SCIENTIFIC FASTING

Other similar **INDIGO BOOKS** available (or to be published shortly) are:

AN INTRODUCTION TO YOGA, Annie Besant

OCCULT PRINCIPLES OF HEALTH AND HEALING, Max Heindel

YOUR FORCES AND HOW TO USE THEM, C. D. Larson

KUNDALINI. The Serpent Power, V. G. Rele

ESOTERIC HEALING. The Sacred Art of Healing, Alice Bailey

YOGA. FOR ETERNAL YOUTH, Sri Yogendra

MEDICAL ASTROLOGY. A GUIDE TO HEALING. A TREATISE ON ASTRO-DIAGNOSIS FROM THE HOROSCOPE AND HAND, Max Meindel & A. F. Heindel

HEALING MANTRAS. SACRED WORDS OF POWER, M. N. Dutt

TANTRIC HEALING. THE POWER OF PHYSICAL, SPIRITUAL, AND PSYCHOLOGICAL HEALING, Sadhu Santideva

HYPNOSIS FOR BEGINNERS, Dylan Morgan

For getting information on our forthcoming books please write to us.

SCIENTIFIC FASTING

a programe for conquering disease

BY

L. B. Hazzard

INDIGO BOOKS

AN
INDIGO BOOK
PUBLISHED BY INDIGO BOOKS
Paperback division of
COSMO PUBLICATIONS,
24-B, Ansari Road, Darya Ganj,
New Delhi 110 002, India.

INDIGO BOOKS and
COSMO PUBLICATIONS
are wholly owned subsidiaries of
GENESIS PUBLISHING PVT. LTD.,
New Delhi, India

SCIENTIFIC FASTING
A progrmae for Conquering Disease

First INDIGO Edition 2003

ISBN 81-292-0028-7

PRINTED AND BOUND IN INDIA

Contents

Preface

Nineteen years have elapsed since the author issued her first volume dealing with the prevention and relief of disease through fasting and its accessories. In each of the three succeeding editions details were added, new discoveries recorded, and all facts tending to throw clearer light upon the practical application of what Dr. Edward Hooker Dewey termed the "New Gospel of Health" were fully exploited. In this, the fifth revised and amplified edition of the work, it is hoped that, with greater detail and greater knowledge, still greater lucidity has been given in exposition of the truths that underlie the therapeutic worth and possibilities of the fast.

The book is written primarily for the lay reader. Hence, whenever a surmise is made or an unproved theory advanced, the attitude of the mind of the author regarding it is plainly displayed. Likewise, whenever absolute harmony has been accomplished between theory and fact, no doubt is permitted the reader in statements of truth discovered.

If science is to be defined as knowledge gained and verified by exact observation and correct thinking, the work in hand is purely a scientific record. The human subjects presented to the author for guidance and care have in all instances been those for whom medicine had done its best, or, if you will, its worst. Each case has been carefully observed; its organic condition and capabilities determined as best they might, the patient was fasted, if this procedure were indicated; or his diet was suited to his needs and the limitations of his organs. Therefore the results obtained are offered no misgivings or apologies. In accomplishing her work the author has been handicapped almost at every step by opposition that at times developed into persecution, and this by those who should have been first to welcome the physiological truths which the text promulgates. The research made, especially that which involved post mortem examination, was achieved only through sheer personal determination, assisted by a few broad minds in authority And it is believed that these autopsies are unique in the history of the healing art, for the author knows of no other investigator who has had opportunity thus to connect the organic consequence of disease directly with its origin. Moreover, each body examined was, for more or less lengthy periods before death, free from drug dosage, offering for examination tissues unaffected by recent artificial chemical stimulus or destructive change from similar cause.

Human progress has ever been associated with constant discovery, and it would show not only deficiency in judgment but actual mental incapacity to decry the achievements of earnest and conscientious seekers after truth among men of medicine. The author, however, differs from these scientists in a number of respects, principally because she has always been of the opinion that the outstanding need of humanity is public health education; and, while she has indicated that medicine is finally awake to this need, too many of its practitioners still are devoted to pathological rather than to physiological investigation. Heretofore the day book of the family physician consisted of a record of visits to households for the treatment of measles, scarlet fever, diphtheria, typhoid fever, or malaria. The man was educated to treat disease and knew little of preventive measures, sanitation, hygiene, or diet, nor did his medical curriculum provide such knowledge. Too long has the medical doctor studied disease and death to the exclusion of health and life. Hence again it is stated that, while the facts presented in the text are intended primarily for lay intelligence, yet, since they are in all instances corroborated, earnest investigation should follow on the part of those men of science who are not bound by prejudice to reject every cult not sanctioned by the traditions and doctrines of their own system of practice.

The aim of medical investigation for many years has been largely towards the classification of the symptoms of disease and the segregation of the micro-organisms discovered in its presence. Because of this the medical physician may and often does delay specific treatment until symptoms develop to a point where what he considers an accurate diagnosis may be made. It is not thought that any intelligent mind will differ with the author when she says that the first things to be considered in the sick-room, the first things that the practitioner of natural therapy considers, are the possibility of recovery and the necessity for prompt and efficient action along lines that tend to the eradication of the cause of disease.

The gospel of good health is based upon the principles of prevention of disease, and there will be found in the introduction to the second edition of this work, published in 1908, these words: "No one knows better than the thinking member of the medical profession that the time is at hand when prevention rather than cure will be the keynote of therapeutics." That this prophecy, for such it has proved, is in part realized, is shown in the trend of thought in every recent article on the subject of medical progress in authoritative professional publications. The family physician now is urged to educate his patients and his community in preventive measures, and so to place himself towards his clientele that his chief service will be one of keeping them well rather than one of curing them when ill. This means that medicine, while still recognizing the specialist, also recognizes that the family physician as a class must form the foundation of all true health service, and that he must maintain most intimate relations with those for whom his guidance is required.

This is exactly what the practitioners of natural therapy have been doing for the past half century and more. For they have ever contended that true perception of cause and effect is the mother of the physician, and that in this understanding there can exist no doubt as to remedy. In other words, not man but nature is the doctor, and nature indicates her curative processes in the existing state of disease. And they who follow nature in her physical law further contend that whatever information they acquire of the procedure through which natural curative processes are carried on shall freely be given to their patients, so that in the future the latter may in great measure be relieved of dependency upon professional guidance.

The upbuilding and the maintenance of the human body lie wholly with its individual possessor, and he should be cognizant of its parts and of the conserving tasks which they perform to the uttermost degree of knowledge. Ignorance in these respects is a universal fault resulting from the custom of depending upon others for specialized information. The message contained in the pages that follow, if rightly perceived and executed, in large degree substitutes for a state of blind dependence upon unharmonized fact and theory one of reliance upon self and natural law.

1 *The Pioneers of Therapeutic Fasting*

In this chapter the author proposes to speak of her personal acquaintance and friendship with those two pioneers in the cause of natural therapy whose names and deeds stand forth as do none other by reason of their intellectuality, their courage, and their ability to grasp the fundamental truths which more or less accidentally were revealed to each of them approximately at the same time. The chapter also purposes a short resume of the contribution of the author to therapeutic fasting and of the difficulties and persecution to which she has been subjected.

It is now about half a century since the newspapers of this country were filled with articles dealing with Dr. Henry S. Tanner and his claim that he had gone without food for forty-two days. One of my purposes in writing this chapter is to dissipate the fiction that the fasts that Dr. Tanner undertook were made in order to attract notoriety—for the mere sake of advertisement They were not. Naturally these fasts attracted attention, and such periods of abstention from food still would attract attention were they brought to public notice. But Dr. Tanner had another object in view, and it is best expressed in his own words as contained in a personal letter dated December 28, 1911.

He says: "I really believe that I am entitled to be called the father of therapeutic fasting in this country, for away back in 1877 I had given up hopes of ever regaining what might be called normal health. I was then in Minneapolis in the practice of my profession, and, after a strenuous time with a patient critically ill, I virtually collapsed. I was at such a low ebb physically and mentally at the time that I did not care whether I lived or died, and I determined that, since my drugs gave me no relief, I would starve myself to death ere I again would suffer the physical misery that had been mine for months preceding. I accordingly told Dr. Moyer, my consulting companion, that I would not again eat food until I was dead or recovered in health." It will be remembered that Dr. Tanner was a fully accredited doctor of medicine.

The facts as recorded are these. On the 15th of July, 1877, Dr. Henry S Tanner was called in consultation with Dr. A. Moyer of Minneapolis, Minnesota, to attend a critical case that detained them late into the night. The next day Dr. Tanner felt ill and did not leave his room. During the day he drank some milk, as he did on the day following. But this was the last food taken by him until August 29th following, a period of forty-two days. Both Dr. Tanner and Dr. Moyer concurred in the opinion that from the viewpoint of medical diagnostics the symptoms in the case were those of low gastric fever. During "treatment"

Dr. Tanner occupied a room in the home of Dr. Moyer, and he was not at any time confined to his bed. He took during the entire forty-two days of abstinence nothing but water into his stomach, but of this he drank freely when thirsty.

At the end of ten days of fasting the symptoms of his disorder disappeared; he gained in strength, and in every way showed physical and mental improvement. Dr. Moyer, however, frequently remonstrated with Dr. Tanner for pursuing what he, Dr. Moyer, believed to be a suicidal course, but Dr. Tanner persisted, and we have in the small volume, *Forty Days Without Food,* a record of the full fast from Dr. Moyer's pen. The latter says, after detailing the daily experiences of his "patient" for forty days:

"The case continued until I became alarmed, and I strenuously urged Dr. Tanner to allay his gastric irritation by taking milk, which he finally consented to do. The next forenoon—that of the forty-second day of fasting—he ate a cracker and drank some lemonade, but this his stomach rejected." In the light of more recent knowledge of the therapeutics of fasting this experience was to be expected. But later on the same day Dr. Tanner went downtown, and, coming home within half an hour, said to Dr. Moyer, "Well, Doctor, I think I have finished affairs for good. I not only have taken a pint of milk, but have eaten five pears and half a good-sized watermelon."

No records were kept either by Dr. Tanner or Dr.

Moyer of the phenomena of this fast. The only data extant deal with the prompt and general relief of symptoms of distress, all of which vanished by the tenth day of fasting, and there is mention made that Dr. Tanner had no passage from the bowels from the 15th of July until the 31st of August, an interval of 47 days. To carry out a fast today in this manner would be deemed a bid for disaster, hence the record made by Dr. Tanner in this, his first essay into prolonged abstinence from food for health's sake, is thus rendered the more remarkable.

The fast in question was commenced with a view of relieving an inflammation of the stomach, and it was continued after the active symptoms had subsided in order to test the worth of scientific teachings as to the time a human being might live without food. No plan had been arranged, for, as stated, decision to fast came suddenly; neither was there any intention of bringing the matter to public attention.

But the outcome of Dr. Tanner's experiment was so surprising and so successful from the therapeutic viewpoint that Dr. Moyer was unable to remain silent, and he told a few of his friends, among whom was a reporter of the *St. Paul Pioneer Press.* This virtually necessitated a public statement of the facts, which called wide-spread attention to Dr. Tanner, and newspapers throughout the country were soon publishing articles and interviews, many of which attempted to throw doubt upon the doctor's veracity. Medical men especially, almost to a man, when questioned upon the subject, stated that such a fast was a physical impossibility, and medical journals published such statements as scientific facts.

These attacks upon Dr. Tanner's probity he believed were likely to affect his professional reputation, and he thereupon determined to speak for himself. This he did through the columns of the *Pioneer Press* in an article iterating what has been related, together with other announcements and arguments that need not here be quoted.

For some time after publication of this communication considerable interest was shown, especially in the Middle West, upon the subject of fasting, not, however, because of its therapeutic possibilities, but because of the doubt that a human being might emulate the Christ and perform in the flesh a miracle. For Christ's fast of forty days and nights was then as now by orthodox believers numbered among miraculous events.

Dr. Tanner went further than this in later years, and, as he says in a letter to the author of date February 23, 1912: "My second fast, publicly given, was called the 'Great American Sensation', and its novel incidents were wired to the ends of the telegraphic world. My advisers planned for me wisely. My object was not money, but to relieve myself of the odium unjustly heaped upon me by the medical enemies of all righteousness. Right triumphed, and the very javelins of hate hurled at me, in their recoil held up the medical profession to the derision of the world. Every prediction of failure was nullified, and I came off conqueror and more than conqueror, in spite of the medical Goliaths arrayed against truth."

This statement was made by Dr. Tanner thirty-two years after he underwent his famous second fast in the City of New York. The fast began on June 28,1880, and ended at noon, August 6,1880, full forty days.

To go into the controversies that this public demonstration occasioned would be futile here. It is sufficient to say that Dr. Tanner successfully vindicated his cause, and that he proved his contention that mere man might refrain from eating for forty days and still live. In addition, he showed that the physical state of his body was materially improved by his experience, and that the therapeutic value of abstinence from food was an established fact. As a result of this test Dr. Tanner's name became a household word, and to this day in works not allied at all to the subject references are met with the good old doctor as their theme.

Dr. Henry S. Tanner was born in England in 1831. He died in San Diego, California, in comparative obscurity in 1919. Eighty-eight years of life, most of which was devoted to contending with the orthodox members of his profession! Yet he never lost his mental poise nor his well developed sense of humor. Nor did he ever descend to the meannesses of petty controversy, although outspoken to the end. Throughout his practice, and he was always actively engaged in the work of his profession, he decried the use of drugs, depending entirely upon natural therapy. When his purse was full, his funds were at the disposal of those in need, and his whole personality was one that carried with it and expressed the Golden Rule.

Dr. Tanner, from 1877 on, employed the fast in his practice. He slightly antedates Dr. Edward Hooker Dewey in this regard, but he did not, as did Dr. Dewey, make of his knowledge the basis of a cult, the foundation of a school.

When in 1911 the author was persecuted by the political members of the orthodox branch of medicine, and was accused of having caused the death of one of her fasting patients by starvation, Dr. Tanner rose to the occasion, as evidenced in the following letter: "Our local papers have published matter in regard to you professionally. As I am the father of fasting, I'm an interested party in your welfare. If I can be of service, command me, and to the extent of my ability to help, I will cheerfully respond."

One could not ask for more than this, yet Dr. Tanner did more. Testimony from witnesses not directly connected with the case was barred at the trial by a prejudiced judge, so it was not possible to take advantage of the doctor's offer at this time. But later, while the case was pending in the higher courts, Doctor Tanner came to Seattle, and he and the author appeared many times jointly on the platform to the great good of the cause of therapeutic fasting. He was then eighty-one years of age and in possession of all of his faculties, save that he was slightly deaf. Upon his return to Los Angeles, where he then made his home, he continued practicing "natural methods" under medical license.

Dr. Tanner died of sheer old age in 1919 at San Diego. It is a sad resection upon those who should have felt the obligation, that the last days of this gentle but firm-principled man should have been spent in the County Hospital. The author had been absent abroad for nearly four years and had lost touch with the doctor, only to discover on her return to this country after his death the facts as here recorded. Eighty-eight years of existence, forty-two of which were devoted to the advancement of that method of healing by which his own life had been saved and prolonged, and devoted as well to teaching others the natural way to health, with what far reaching effects none of us may ever know! In that he advocated and practiced fasting and other natural therapeutic measures for the long space of forty-two years, and that he was first to attract public attention to the possibilities of the fast as a curative means, to Dr. Henry S. Tanner is justly entitled the first place among the pioneers of therapeutic fasting.

Just about the time that Dr. Tanner in Minneapolis discovered for himself the worth of abstinence from food as a therapeutic measure, another medical physician in Meadville, Pennsylvania, by what may be called pure accident, was given a revelation of the power of nature in disease along lines similar to the Tanner experience. Wonder is occasioned at the coincidence in time and in circumstance. Dr. Tanner says definitely that his first trial of the fast was a personal and experimental one, and that he began his initial experience on the 17th day of July, 1877. Dr. Edward Hooker Dewey, on page 48 of his *True Science of Living,* states: "On a hot day in July, 1877, I entered a home to assume charge of a case of typhoid fever that was to arouse every possible faculty as by an electric charge." The doctor began to treat this case in orthodox medical manner, and in order to support strength and vital power, from the medical viewpoint it was his duty to enforce feeding. But, fortunately for the patient and for the future of scientific fasting in disease, every dose of drugs or of food, every drink of water, was instantly rejected by the stomach, and this condition persisted for over three weeks. In this connection Dr. Dewey remarks: "I was a very surprised physician, for, even without food, I found the tongue cleaning and a manifest gain in both mental and physical strength that became even marked at the time, when, to my continued surprise, food might be borne. I, however, determined to let nature continue to have her way, and from the end of the third week I watched, without trying enforced feeding, until the thirty-fourth day, when my patient, with natural hunger in evidence, began to eat and to rebuild with ultimate return to normal vigor.

"Here," he continues, "was an object lesson:

"(1) Vital power supported without food.

"(2) Mental and physical strength increasing with

the decline of symptoms.

"(3) A cure without the aid of remedies, and one that was eminently complete in every way.

"(4) No unusual wasting of the body."

In later years, when relating his early experiences in connection with fasting in disease, Dr. Dewey, both in conversation and in writing, dwelt at great length upon the complete reversal of personal opinion and belief which the conditions and the outcome of this case produced. He gives in detail in his several books the results of this change of thought, and the tale is as interesting as is one of adventure or romance, for it led this man into life-long advocacy and practice of a method diametrically opposed to that for which he had been trained, and which he had theretofore made his profession. It also brought to him controversy, ridicule, and persecution.

He who becomes a renegade from an established creed is more than likely to find himself an outcast from the society of believers in that creed. And Dr. Dewey, once launched upon a course which he deemed that of the truth, proved no exception to the common fate. His medical confreres at first dubbed him eccentric—even crazy. And it was not long before his presence in consultation and in professional assemblage was no more desired. In fact, the local medical society requested his resignation as a member of its body. But Dr. Dewey possessed among other sterling qualities, courage, and he never wavered, but sturdily and steadily continued in his chosen path until recognition of his discovery and of his teachings was forced, first upon his clientele, and then upon his colleagues, by the results which his methods obtained.

Dr. Dewey is perhaps best known to the world as the strenuous advocate of the "No Breakfast Plan", and his book with this title has circled the globe. But his other works, notably *The True Science of Living,* well bear careful reading, even though in the light of later and more scientific investigation discovery, his theory and practice of the fast leave many things to be supplied.

It is not, however, the purpose of the author to write in criticism of the work of the pioneers in the art and science of physiatrics, for it is sufficient that these men first made exposition of present-day natural practice, later to be developed and elaborated by their disciples. And it is also to be remembered that, as is the destiny of every pioneer, they proved no exception to the rule, and were reviled and persecuted exquisitely by those who should have supported their investigations, those who should have worked out with them the possibilities of their discoveries. Entrenched authority invariably escapes ridicule and persecution, since in most instances it is individually devoid of acumen and initiative, and is smugly content to dwell within the vicious thrall of orthodoxy.

Dr. Dewey was born at Wayland, Pennsylvania, in May, 1839. In the late fifties he entered thc employ of a local druggist, and he spent two years dispensing remedies and absorbing pharmaecopoeial lore. He says for himself that at that time he came into contact with all kinds of physicians and with all kinds of "isms" in medical practice, and that the prescription counter is a wonderful revelator of the literary and scientific attainments of the medical profession, yet it fails to account for the relative degree of success of men who are without the slightest shade of scientific conception of the action of a remedy or of its indicated need as revealed by symptoms. He further says that his drugstore experience led to a slowly developing conviction that, as an adaptation of means to an end, the administration of drugs for the cure of disease is one of the most unscientific of human vocations. It is evident that this conviction did not then become an entity in the doctor's mind, for it did not deter him from going. ahead with those studies that finally brought him to the College of Medicine and Surgery of the University of Michigan. From this college he was graduated in 1864 with a medical degree, and almost immediately we find him as an acting assistant surgeon in the army of the United States on duty at a field hospital at Chattanooga, Tennessee. When discharged at the close of the war, the doctor chose Meadville, Pennsylvania, as his field of labor, and in the autumn of 1866 he became a general practitioner in that small city, then numbering about ten thousand souls. Here for eleven years he followed the paths of orthodoxy, still with that slowly developing conviction disturbing his professional thought, until, as has been related, in 1877 sudden light was given and his conviction, now confirmed, became the guiding principle of the remainder of his life.

Thenceforth Dr. Dewey was eminently successful in a practice based upon causing his patients to abstain from food for periods short or long; upon inaugurating the no-breakfast plan; and upon impressing upon his followers in illness and in health the beneficent effects of fresh air, pure water, and sunshine. But, as has been indicated, there was much in the fundamentals of his method that needed revision, and he was lamentably lacking, as was Dr. Tanner, in perceiving that prompt and efficient auxiliary hygienic means must constantly be employed while the extreme process of elimination occasioned by a fast is in progress. He repudiated the use of the enema or internal bath, and preferred and insisted upon waiting upon the bowels to act "naturally", as he termed it. In later years, when the writer enrolled as a student with Dr. Dewey, her own thought led her first to suggest and then to remonstrate upon this and other vital omissions in procedure, and at one time only her friendship for her preceptor prevented a break in relations. It was not until a few months before Dr. Dewey died that he partially acknowledged his error in these respects and deplored the fact that he had continually advised against the use of the enema, which he had finally come to recognize as the most essential of hygienic accessories connected with a scientifically conducted fast.

The physiology of abstinence from food for the prevention and relief of disease as determined by Dr.

Dewey and published to the world in his books is beyond all doubt correct. But the doctor was much astray in the hygiene necessary to the successful issue of therapeutic fasting. Accepting neither the eliminative assistance of the enema nor that of daily cleansing the surface of the body, he ignored as well the dietetic requisites, both preparatory and subsequent to the total abstinence interval. And as to diet in health, the doctor exhibited the common failing of the medical profession, which then as now seems to consider food merely as fuel for the body, with but little regard for its digestibility or its nutritive content.

Dr. Dewey died from paralysis, a condition that arose solely from error in personal dietary. He conscientiously observed the "no breakfast plan," which he advised for others, but food values, food adaptability, food combination, all were ignored in the two daily meals he permitted himself. Meats and fish, eggs and milk, breads and pastries, with comparatively few vegetables in combination, and these mostly of the starchier kinds, formed his food supply. What wonder that hardened veins, high blood pressure, and ultimate paralysis developed!

Dr. Dewey suffered his first stroke of apoplexy on March 28, 1904. For sixteen days he fasted and gradual improvement took place, so much so, that in several months he again became active in his profession. At that time the author was most desirous that the doctor accept her proved conclusions concerning the internal bath and the dietary essential when a fast is broken. But to no avail, and her warning went for a time unheeded, until untoward symptoms again arising, Dr. Dewey consented to close his practice and to come to Minneapolis there to be under the care and direction of his erstwhile pupil. He was delayed in departure, and a second paralytic seizure occurred on December 10, 1904, resulting in his death on the 21st of the same month.

In personal contact with Dr. Dewey and in a voluminous correspondence he ever dwelt with great inspiration and broad vision upon what he called "New Gospel of Health", emphasizing at all times the thought that the lesson he was endeavoring to impart was one that applied to every human ill. He said so often that he wanted me clearly to see, as he did, the divine hand in cure through an evolution in reverse. By this he meant that disease in the structural changes involved is a matter of nature's own work—just as clearly as in those structural changes by which the body was originally developed. And he further added that the cure of disease is but an analogous process in reverse of its cause. This reasoning is clear and logical, and its conclusions are truth.

Dr. Dewey is dead, but his work lives, and, because his was a mind of system and of science, the foundation he laid for the new gospel of health, which nevertheless is the oldest of hygienic truths because it is nature's own system of law, will stand for all time. Natural therapy owes to Dr. Edward Hooker Dewey both recognition and honor as the first scientifically able pioneer in the field of therapeutic fasting.

Since the remainder of the chapter in hand deals with the personal work of the author, she will, it is hoped, be pardoned for speaking in the first person.

My work in natural therapy dates back nearly thirty years, to July, 1898, to be exact. As did Dr. Tanner, I arrived at my preliminary knowledge by way of illness. My girlhood, which was spent in the lake region of Minnesota, was given over to a healthful, athletic life, filled with every sort of outdoor exercise and work. My mother, who never touched animal food in her life, possessed a knowledge of dietetic combinations and of cookery, which was purely instinctive, since there were no opportunities cast her way for its acquirement. In consequence the family table was supplied mostly with food vegetarian in character. My father, who was of similar habit and belief, unfortunately at about the time I was seven years old, so far compromised with his principles as to employ a medical physician upon a yearly basis to care for the family health. This physician was convinced, as were the majority of his profession at that day, that all children harbored intestinal parasites, and that periodic doses of some vermifuge were essential. Therefore I, in company with my brothers and sisters, was given some blue mass pills, a strong mercurial preparation. I now allow, what of course I could not then suspect, that this powerful poison did irreparable injury to my intestines, retarding and preventing their development and growth to such degree that even to this day I am compelled to resort to the enema daily.

After the blue mass experience, for a long time I was never well. No diet, however carefully chosen, agreed with me, and life thereafter during the rest of my childhood and well into young womanhood became a dreary search for health. In this search I learned much of what was then taught concerning dietetics both from orthodox and unorthodox sources, but no permanent relief was ever vouchsafed me until in 1898 I heard of the work and the remarkable successes of Dr. Dewey. As a result of the inspiration I thus received, with some trepidation I attempted a fast, and went four days without food. A little later I dared still more and tried fasting for one whole week, with benefits that were so pronounced that whatever reservations I may have felt vanished completely. Since then I have fasted many times, and, when necessary, for longer periods. And I attribute the robust health which now is mine as well as the comparatively lengthy span of years I have attained to the practice of what I preach, to the taking of my own medicine.

Shortly after I began to take practical interest in fasting I made the acquaintance of Dr. Dewey, and at his invitation I placed myself under his tutelage. I was then studying osteopathy, but, after a term spent under the instruction of Dr. Dewey, and with my own fasting experience to guide me, I became convinced that osteopathy alone was not the panacea its advocates claimed, but I believed, as I still believe, that in conjunction with other remedial measures, among which dieting and fasting are of most import, its therapeutic value might be greatly increased. And I have found this so.

In Minneapolis, where I first located, my early practice proved a struggling one, but gradually I had the satisfaction of seeing it grow steadily and surely, for the results that accrued from my then rather drastic application of the complete fast were such as to surprise Dr. Dewey as well as myself. Cases pronounced incurable by medical physicians recovered under the regimen I imposed, and the symptoms presented ranged from chronic constipation, diabetes, Bright's disease, and syphilis to paralysis. Called to the Pacific Coast in 1906, I decided there to remain, and in the summer of that year I opened offices in Seattle. Soon after this I began to encounter organized persecution from medical sources, aided by newspapers controlled by the profession. Such deaths as occurred under my care received the widest publicity, and the accounts written concerning them were distorted and filled with implication, innuendo, and threat. These articles eventually accomplished the end sought by their authors, for in 1912 I was brought to trial charged with having willfully caused the death of an English woman patient through starvation.

A jury divided amongst itself, but urged to decision by a prejudiced judge and by public sentiment inflamed by a public press, determined that my crime was that of manslaughter, and I was thereupon sentenced to a minimum term of two years in the penitentiary. I served these years day by day in anguish of body and of mind, until finally the then Governor of Washington became convinced of my innocence and of the monstrous injustice that had been done, and he granted to me an unconditional pardon, restoring all of the rights and privileges which by reason of my conviction I had forfeited.

In 1916, shortly after my pardon was granted, I was called to New Zealand to take charge of the case of a friend, and I spent nearly four years in that country, every day of the time devoted to a large and successful practice. But home ties and home duties brought me back to the home land, and here I continue the work with bettered surroundings, increased facilities, and with perspective and concept broadened by experiences to which those of my predecessors and contemporaries compare as mere bagatelles.

Because of my intimate association with Dr. Dewey in the early years of my work, because he deemed me a practitioner worthy of his confidence during his last hours, and because I have developed to the utmost his theory and his art, I do not think that I can be denied my place with him and with Dr. Tanner as a pioneer in the therapeusis of the fast.

There are others, physicians as well as laymen, to whom is due recognition as pioneers in furthering the fast as a remedial measure. Among these must be mentioned Charles C. Haskell, now deceased, also a writer and issuer of books, who was friend of Dr. Dewey and his publisher as well; Lloyd Jones, head of the firm of H.

I. Jones & Son, Ltd., book dealers and publishers, of Wanganui, New Zealand, whose personal advocacy, writings and publications have done so much to spread the new gospel of health throughout Australia and the South Seas; and the late Dr. C. E. Page of Boston. All of these are entitled to place and honor for their untiring efforts in support of the doctrine promulgated in the pages of the text.

Unity of Disease and Cure 2

Fasting and Starvation Defined: Distinction between Functional and Organic Disease: The Cause of Impure Blood: The Nature of Disease and Cure

Disease and cure are a unity. The former may not be suppressed lest the latter fail of attainment. In order that a clear conception of the substance of the text may be obtained, a short explanation of the meaning of the thought expressed in the first sentence and of the principles upon which the efficacy of the fast in the treatment of disease is based is essential. It is also necessary, for the purpose of defining the distinction that exists between fasting and starvation, to discuss later on the physiological changes developed in the progress of the latter phenomenon, since, in the popular mind, fasting is invariably confounded with starvation.

Fasting is defined as follows:—the voluntary denial of food to a system which is diseased, and which, because of disease, neither demands nor desires nourishment until, rested, purified, and with hunger in evidence, it is again able to resume its metabolic processes. Then, and not till then, is food supplied; then, and not till then, does starvation begin.

For the purposes of the text starvation is defined as the denial of food, by accident or design, to a system needing and demanding sustenance. Hunger, true desire for food, indicates the want and calamitous consequences ensue when its call is denied.

Relieving physical unbalance by voluntarily withholding food is based upon the logical conclusion of the argument herein that, disregarding the variously designated symptoms by which disease is manifested in differing subjects, always there is present one predominating morbid phenomenon—an impure blood current. And the cause of impure blood is primarily faulty nutrition.

An important distinction in condition here needs exposition. Organic disease, whether inherent, or the result of continued functional disturbance, or of physical shock, is that in which one or more of the organs of the body is deformed, undeveloped, or otherwise structurally disabled so as to interfere with its work, a state comparable to that of a machine with a defective cog.

Functional disease is that in which the vital organs in general are in condition to do their work, but certain of them have become unable partially or wholly to function by reason of congestion and irritation, the result of food chemically changed into noxious substances through causes later to be related in detail. In this state fermentation and putrefaction occur in the intestinal canal and elsewhere, and toxins are produced that enter the blood, thus impairing its quality and deranging the vital processes. Extra labor is also entailed upon other organs, since they are not only stimulated in unwonted degree by the presence of substances harmful to their action, but are also compelled to perform, in so far as they may, the work of their disabled allies.

Organic disease is a cause in itself of faulty nutrition, for, when it is present, the organs affected are always partially crippled in function. While this form of disease is usually beyond the hope of recovery, its harmful results may be reduced to a minimum by means of judicious application of the fast at properly regulated intervals; and a combination of abstinence from food with corrective dieting will lengthen the life of the sufferer to the degree to which a defective organism will permit vitality to operate.

Functional disease and its ultimate consequence, functionally caused organic disease, are the results of nutrition impaired by incorrect methods in feeding, by improper selection of food, or by a supply beyond the power of the metabolic processes to handle. The latter include those operations by which on the one hand dead food is converted into living tissue, and on the other by which living matter is broken down into simpler products in a cell or organism. In any of the circumstances poisons are produced that injure the system, until finally the condition becomes general and disease is apparent. The subject cannot have been ignorant of disturbance for some time previous to actual disability, for minor aches and pains have given ample warning. Mild preventive steps, taken when symptoms first appear, will obviate by anticipative action later drastic measures, but natural resident power of contending against bodily abuse is limited only by individual characteristics, and these may permit of extended transgression of hygienic law. Usually a positive halt is not called until the physical machinery has been well nigh obstructed with food waste and its products

It is possible that at first sight the principles here set forth may not be fully apprehended, hence, as important premises to the argument, they are again enumerated for reference by the student in connection with the body of the text.

In disease, whatever abnormal conditions are present, whatever the nominal symptom, an impure blood stream is always discovered.

Impure blood is caused primarily by impaired nutrition.

Impaired nutrition results from

(a) Taking into the body food wrongly selected in kind or in quantity, wrongly prepared, or wrongly masticated.

(b) Taking into the body food that may have been correctly selected, prepared, and eaten, but that in quantity is greater than is needed for the repair and growth of tissue.

(c) Nerve force inhibited at its source, at some point in transmission, or by reflexive stimulus, irritation, at its termini.

(d) Mental perturbation, such as worry, fear, jealousy, anger, and the like.

Any of these causes being operative, food ingested fails of complete digestion, ferments and putrefies, generating circulating poison that creates and continues disease until the producing cause can be eliminated.

Inherent or congenital organic disease and functionally caused organic disease in its later stages embody defects in form, size, or cell structure of any one of the vital organs. Except in rare instances through surgical intervention, such structural deficiencies are beyond the hope of repair, but a carefully selected dietary combined with judicious application of the fast and its accessories will afford relief and prolong existence.

In disease that is purely functional in cause the vital organs are normally developed and are physically perfect in structure, but are obstructed in action by food-excess and its toxic products. Functionally caused disease is a condition that always admits of full recovery, and cure is a certainty when natural law is permitted its course.

Any symptom of disease is evidence of poison circulating in the blood. The conventional method of treatment invariably aims at the suppression of the symptom rather than at the removal of its cause. On the other hand, the natural manner of handling the situation recognizes disease as health perverted, and far from attempting to suppress its symptoms it aims at still further uncovering the condition by assisting the action of the very evident eliminative process in operation. And oftentimes this assistance of the eliminative function results in an aggravation of symptoms, in an apparent increase in the severity of disease. This is a purely logical and salutary consequence of natural curative phenomena. Disease in itself being but a process of the elimination of toxins from the system, nature, given free rein, thus expresses herself in determined effort towards the restoration of health, the normal state of physical existence

Hunger and disease cannot exist simultaneously in the animal body. This is a truth that cannot be too strongly emphasized. When hunger is absent because of disease, food is required neither for cell rebuilding nor for strength, and all animate creation, save man, obeys the primal law of abstinence when the physical scale no longer balances. Knowing that disease arises from a single source, natural therapeutics knows as well but a single means of relief—rest for organs overworked, and prompt removal by natural aids of substances deleterious to health.

To revert to the symptoms of disease—the function of digestion is generally regarded as an extensive and complicated process, and it is so closely related to the functions of other parts of the body that it is difficult to describe the bounds, if any, beyond which digestion has no influence. The digestive apparatus is commonly spoken of as including the alimentary canal and those important glands that contribute secretions to the successive processes involved; but, as absorption and assimilation, on the one hand, and formation and withdrawal of waste products, on the other, are so nearly related to preliminary digestion, it is impossible to form a clear conception of disease of the digestive organs, for instance, without observing the state of other and contributory parts of the body. While it makes for simplicity of description to exclude those organs not commonly grouped with the digestive apparatus, this does not result in a correct understanding, and therefore, if an explanation is to be found, not only for a disturbed physiological state, but also, in instances, for structural changes in the digestive organs, the field must be widened, and study be directed to the nervous system, including its physical manifestations, to the fluids of the body, to the rebuilding and breaking-down of tissue, and to the eliminative functions as well. Unconsciously a great part of the importance of this general view is perhaps recognized when it is assumed that good digestion depends upon restful sleep, fresh air, sunlight, physical exercise, and activity of the bowels, kidneys, and skin. But, disregarding these essential matters, it is difficult to apprehend the nature of digestive disturbances, or to prescribe for their relief. It may truly be said of an individual that, in a sense, his digestive ailment arises in the brain, in the lungs, in the heart, or in the kidneys, but the distinctions and differences stated must be clearly kept in mind lest the idea of the unity of disease and cure be clouded. It must be fully understood that the study of disease of the stomach is not limited to that organ, that the symptom expressed is merely that of disturbances that may be widely distributed throughout the body. Medicine has sought to give disease names that are specifically classified, names based upon the locality of expression of the symptom; but this, it is seen, is only a relatively justifiable conception. There are no symptoms referable solely to the kidneys, to the heart, to the blood; the man is sick from a single cause; his illness appears here or there, but his body is sick as a whole.

It is surprising to discover that the disturbances of the functions of the human body should not long since have been traced to their single source. Long ago should pain and other distressing symptoms of illness have been recognized as benevolent warnings, sharp reminders of a condition, not perhaps yet fully developed, but as warnings that in themselves should compel the repose that is necessary, and that should forbid admission into the body of substances that are injurious.

The doctrine of unity in the cause and cure of disease as set forth in the text of this work has been carefully and earnestly investigated by the author through a period of more than thirty years. Thousands of cases have been treated upon this basis, and each instance has but confirmed the conviction that the principle involved is absolutely sound. It has stood all tests. When death during a fast has occurred, the autopsy invariably revealed organic deficiency, inherent or acquired through years of continuous functional abuse. But in all cases of disease purely functional in cause, proper application of the method led to complete recovery.

So far as may be accomplished in a work of this size, the fast as a therapeutic agency, with its effects both upon the body and mind, is fully discussed. What is asked of the reader is that he lay aside prejudice and approach the subject without bias, keeping before the eyes of his mind the words of the apostle:—"Prove all things; hold fast that which is good."

Starvation 3

Starving from Overfeeding: There is no Hunger when Disease is Manifest

The chief purpose of food is that of supplying the tissue of the body with the elements necessary for its growth and maintenance. In the event that, through faulty digestion, through organic defect, or through deficiency in the functions of absorption and assimilation, tissue waste is not replaced as broken down, starvation ensues. In any of the designated conditions, the more food supplied, the less resistance to disease succeeds since energy then must be directed to the elimination of food and food products that cannot be utilized because of physical inability in the ultimate processes, and finally exhaustion and death occur.

Dr. E. H. Dewey said, "The body may be well fed but still be starving to death." This statement may be made more striking and perhaps more lucid by saying that in reality it is the overfed body that is continuously in a starving condition, and this by a process that is much more distressing in effect than is that by which death is caused when food is indefinitely denied. And starving of this sort, starving from overfeeding, is well nigh the universal manner in which the individual existence of man is terminated, for every symptom of disease, every disease epidemic, owes its development to food wrongly combined, and ingested always in excess, and usually far in excess, of body requirement, with malnutrition as its consequence.

Each cell that enters the structure of the human organism may be regarded as an entity, as an individual life center, with power to select and to appropriate for its maintenance suitable constructive material from the blood current, and with power to eliminate its own waste. This being true, the life of the body as a whole is reflected in miniature in each of its cells, the infinitesimal particles that go to form its structure. In health, when equilibrium is sustained between nutrition and elimination, every cell capably performs its function, receives its needful quota of pabulum, and discharges its waste. In disease the condition changes. Material then absorbed is the product of ill-digested or non-digested food, elimination is also at fault, and the cell finds its source of maintenance, the blood stream, vitiated. For a time the small body is supported by its inherent vitality and by its stored food reserve, but, if proper nourishment is denied, if the condition of toxemia persists, it atrophies and eventually dies. The death of cells sufficient in number to cause a vital organ to fail in function causes the death of the body. And thus, in a sense, it may be said that all animal dissolution, exclusive of that caused by accident, is brought about through starvation

The usual concept of starvation is that the body perishes for some reason or other because it is not supplied with food for its maintenance and growth. But elements and conditions other than those caused by deprivation of food enter into starving to death, for the latter cannot occur in ordinary circumstances, as the text demonstrates, within a few days or weeks, or even months, when the resources of the body have been in any degree conserved.

In a scientifically conducted fast death from starvation cannot take place when organic disease is absent. In every animate body a reserve supply of nourishment is held in the interstices of tissue. Brain and nerves are at all times directly supported by this stored food, and, when wounds, sores, or fractures of bone call for repair, a healthy surplus furnishes the demand. Not until this reserve is exhausted or prevented from being appropriated by nerve structure can death intervene.

When disease is manifest, there is no hunger—there cannot be, for the body then indicates through physical distress first, that it desires functional rest, and next, that it is in process of relieving itself of the cause of its distress. And, until its purposes are accomplished, vitality is more weakly expressed, since the paths for the transfer of energy are largely obstructed. But the vehicle of vitality, the organism itself, is conserved for a time by means of its sinking-fund of nourishment. If by continued feeding—and any feeding in disease is pernicious—the avenues for the expression of life force are further obstructed, strength finally may be no longer manifested, and death will occur. On the other hand, when nature is permitted full scope, the cause of disease is eliminated, and true hunger appears. Then, with food supplied, rebuilding and growth are resumed in a system purified and functionally equal to its appointed tasks.

The law of hunger, the primal rule of being in animal existence, is reserved for discussion later in the text. It is the safeguard of bodily resource, and its claims may never be ignored.

Disease may be induced through the action of mental states upon physical function, and in accidental conditions that compel abstinence from food, such as shipwreck, mine disasters, and the like, digestive function is paralyzed by mental apprehension. If death should occur in these circumstances, within a comparatively short time, it must be attributed, not to lack of nourishment, but to the effect of fear, of general emotional exhaustion, upon physical forces.

It is an error to associate the terms, fasting and starvation. Fasting conduces to systemic purification; starvation is actual systemic poisoning. One may and often does starve on three full daily meals. And it may be added that it requires great skill to fast an individual properly, but that any tyro can starve a man to death.

When and Why to Fast 4

The Time to Fast is When One is Ill: The Body Gets Sick as a Whole: General Hints about Fasting

Fasting is indicated only when illness impends or is in actual evidence. No need exists in health for the employment of measures for the alleviation of pain and distress for these signs are non-evident when physical balance is the rule. Remedial means are necessary only in illness, impending or actual, and then alone should the fast and its accessories be applied.

In disease nature is in process of purifying the body—is casting out its waste, thus cleansing the system in preparation for active, healthy rebuilding. The fast as an eliminative measure is comparable to no other agency known, but before entering upon a period of abstinence from food, the subject, whether under guidance or conducting his own case, should fully comprehend the details of the truth that physical lack of balance is due to a single cause. The symptoms that then are present, or that may arise thereafter during the fast or upon a dietary regimen, need occasion no alarm, for their source is understood and their meaning is rightly conceived as therapeutic in character. Omission of food permits the eliminative organs to act unhampered by intake, and in this omission and in the employment the essential hygienic accessories is discovered the sole means of assistance that will assure permanent relief. Alleviation of symptomatic distress may, however, be accomplished locally through simple measures—dry heat, hot fomentations, cold applications, sunlight, fresh air, body manipulation, vertebral adjustment, and the baths and the enema.

Illness never occurs at the convenient moment. Its warnings may develop in any season of the year, and they should promptly be heeded regardless of personal inconvenience or of climatic situation. To wait until disease develops locally is always disastrous, and in the therapeutics of nature diagnosis is unnecessary, for natural measures for relief in any and all illness are identical in essence, varying only in minor details. During a fast, because of the absence of food stimulation, of the heat-producing chemical reactions normal to health, the body is easily chilled, hence it is at times suggested that the fast wait for the warm weather of summer. But, again, the time to fast is when ill, and one should never be deterred from undergoing treatment because the season is not propitious. Artificial means of maintaining indoor temperature are always available, and the needful hygienic requirements may be utilized with equal facility and success whether outer air be warm or cold.

It is to be noted that the winter season is nature's time of rest and recuperation. Then trees and plants are dormant, many animals hibernate, and all nature prepares for the growing period, the resurrection of the spring. Man, because of artificial environment and custom, and with the thought that the body heat is derived solely from fuel consumed, from food ingested, eats more heavily in winter and approaches spring with a system overloaded with waste. Spring fever and spring tonic are reciprocating terms, and epidemic disease is more prevalent then than at any other season.

The symptoms by which disease is exhibited may be specifically named and classified—it may be said that the subject suffers from Bright's disease, from eczema, from diphtheria, or from small-pox, but behind the symptom lies the cause, and, as before stated, the body is not to be thought of as ill in a specific locality or in an individualized organ. It is sick as a whole, though the signs of physical unbalance are more visible, more severely expressed, in one part or another. Illness results when equilibrium no longer exists between nutrition and elimination, resulting in a blood current vitiated at its source, powers of resistance lowered, and soil for germs produced. One remedy alone may cope with this condition, and it is that which nature indicates and employs—elimination of the toxins that cause disease, and rest for organs that have been functioning under stress.

Nature inevitably focuses her efforts at cure upon the point or points of least resistance, upon those outlets of the body that are least able to withstand the pressure exerted to expel material noxious to the system. In health the latter is discharged through those channels that are especially designed for the purpose. The simplest forms in which illness is manifested are colds, headaches, and rashes that appear upon the skin. Because of injudicious feeding, of congestion and overwork, the digestive organs are hampered in function. Elimination through bowels, kidneys, lungs, and skin is naturally continued to the limit of the power of these organs. When any one of them is overtaxed, a portion of its labor is necessarily thrown upon the others. They respond, and in responding they too show distress. When the skin is thus called upon for work beyond its limitations, pimples or rashes appear on its surface. Likewise when the breathing apparatus labors with excess of toxic matter, the latter appears as a discharge from the mucus membrane of the throat and the nose, and, if these organs are unable to cope with their unaccustomed task, the lungs in turn are called upon, and, unless speedily relieved, they become clogged and inflamed, a condition dangerous in the extreme. Normally equal balance should exist among all of the organs of elimination. Each should perform its allotted task proportionately with the others. The arms of the scale of intake and outgo should constantly remain at level, and this they do when health is the rule.

The social surroundings of a fasting patient are of the utmost import. The effect of mental states upon physical well being will not be dwelt upon here, but, when friends and family object to the administration of a fast, their opposition is more than apt to be the cause of an emotional crisis. These objections are mainly made because of lack of knowledge of the purpose of the fast and of the details of its application. Ignorant of the principle that underlies this wholly natural agency for the cure of disease, its outcome is feared, and, while the patient is ready and willing to submit to the regimen imposed, relatives and friends may resist to the point of compulsion. Since peace of mind and quiet environment are essential, in these circumstances separation from anxious but misguided intimates is virtually indispensable to favorable result.

Worry, anger, grief, and other morbid emotions are also most detrimental to progress towards cure. One instance comes to mind of a case that had fasted but eight days for functional disease of no especial gravity. Improvement had been continuous, but differences had occurred between the patient and her husband and the latter, in an interview with his wife on the eighth day of her fast, so angered and distressed her that a nervous congestive chill, with suffusion of blood to the brain and lungs resulted, death succeeding. No argument could convince the orthodox mind that the fast was not responsible for the fatal consequence in this case. But the woman would have died just as surely had the scene related taken place before the omission of food, when the patient was physically and nervously weaker than at the time when anger and grief were so strongly excited.

In cases of functional disease, when the patient is not so depleted as to be bedridden, moderate daily exercise during a fast is beneficial. The ordinary duties of life may sometimes be continued with advantage, but, while some fasting subjects may follow their usual vocations, others are compelled to rest throughout the period of abstinence. Usually the greater part of the latter are sufferers from disease either chronically functional or organic in character. Mild mental activity is of value because of the diversion of the mind from contemplation of physical ills. The ideal method in personal conduct during a fast, however, embodies the practice of the sick animal, which remains quiescent, resting absolutely the while it refrains from eating.

It is to be emphasized at this point in the discussion that it is far better that the patient should so occupy himself while fasting that, in so far as is possible, his illness and his treatment be not at any time uppermost in his mind. This is not always a condition easily brought about, for, because of comparatively limited knowledge of the method, the majority of its cases is recruited from the chronically invalided, usually medically treated for years, and accustomed to constant thought of personal pain and distress. It may here be said that the relief occasioned by the fast very often permits these cases in large part to forget their ailments, and to devote their attention to the essentials of living. Occupation and diversion assist materially in accomplishing this result.

In the ordinary case of functional disease the fast

to complete purification is at once suggested. The law of hunger determines its duration, and, all other things being equal, surroundings and mental attitude being in accord, this course will assure restoration to health. When the environment is not congenial, or when, in the opinion of the director of treatment, the condition is such as to require it, a partial fast interrupted by periods of corrective diet, may be used to advantage. Sometimes, too, the facilities for carrying out a complete fast are not afforded, and here the partial or interrupted fast may be deemed a better policy than its finished counterpart. The end is eventually identical, although it is somewhat longer in accomplishment.

There are cases in which the poisonous products of digestive ferment are present in quantity such as to tax the eliminative organs beyond their capability. When this is so, when certain serious and extreme symptoms occur after a fast is begun, these signs are in effect evidences of organic deficiency, and both knowledge and caution are then most necessary in order to carry the case to successful conclusion. Because of the general belief that every symptom is a sign of segregated disease, the average mind has been imbued with the idea that it must regard the symptom to the exclusion of the underlying cause. When, as happens in a fast, a characteristic sign of disease appears in aggravated form after months or years of intermittent occurrence, experience leads to the conclusion that illness is no longer due to simple functional derangement but to actual organic deficiency. Here the partial or interrupted fast is desirable, not because the protracted fast would not accomplish results with better prospect of favorable outcome, but because the patient, no matter how well he may be advised, is apt to fail to appreciate what temporary symptomatic aggravation in the fast implies.

An organ structurally defective cannot be expected to work to full normal capability. Each of the organs of the body will at all times do its utmost, will labor to the limit of its powers, but, forced beyond this limit, it must fail to respond. In cases of this sort, a fast is to be approached with care and intelligence, for only thus may be discovered the organic limitations, the organic deficiencies, of the body in question. During a fast all vital parts are engaged in a supreme process of purification—of casting out the toxic substances that are causing their disease. And, when it is seen through symptoms increased in severity that one or other of these parts is incapable of full duty, the process of elimination is to be assisted by natural stimulation of organs other than the one that is deficient in functioning ability. Such assistance may only be had by the employment of the hygienic accessories later to be described in the text.

Illustrative Cases 5

Fasting Applied to Cases of Inflammatory Rheumatism, Chorea, Epilepsy, Pregnancy, etc.

The Cases dealt with in this chapter are typical but not exhaustive. They are selected from a large number solely because of their representative character, and as evidence that, since the fast is the most effective of all eliminative agents, it reaches indiscriminately but in like manner every phase of functional disability and all organic disease that is not beyond repair. Properly administered, the fast with its accessories insures in all such cases full systemic purification, which is the basis of health.

The first case selected is that of the disease symptom known as inflammatory rheumatism. When first seen the patient, a boy seventeen years of age, was in a precarious state. His condition had been declared by the medical adviser as hopeless, and a limit of twenty-four hours was set within which death must occur. The resources of the physician had been exhausted, and in his opinion all that could be done was to alleviate the excruciating pain with opiates, thus permitting dissolution to take place while the youth was under their influence, and this was the course pursued. The distracted family as a last resort turned to the fast. After examining the case, the writer accepted the responsibility, and a description of the condition of the young man will perhaps throw stronger light upon the contrast that is always displayed between the methods followed by man in disease and those which nature employs.

The boy had been in bed for five weeks; his body showed all of the evidences of the ravages of disease and of those of the remedies that had been applied. The left arm, wrist, and hand were greatly swollen and painful, as were also both knees and ankles. The face was flushed, the breathing stertorous, the pulse very irregular, while the body temperature was 105 degrees. In all respects the working foundation for favorable outcome was most insecure. For two weeks immediately preceding the change in treatment heart action had been stimulated with digitalis and with strychnine; food had been forced upon a protesting stomach as many times daily as the patient could be induced to swallow; and, when the pain had become too severe to be borne, or when delirium occurred, codein and other opiates had been used unsparingly. In addition, within the preceding seven days two quarts of brandy had been poured into the youth. As the result of disease and of drugs the patient could neither lie down nor sit up, and his position was a painful compromise.

Death seemed imminent, but food was at once withheld, and a gentle massage treatment was administered in order to equalize circulation as much as was possible in the circumstances. A half hour after this, an enema of warm water brought away a large amount of fecal matter, all of which resulted in pulse and temperature showing decided downward tendencies, while the patient rested more quietly and easily than for many days.

In acute crises, such as this, drastic measures are imperative, and, on the second day, application of more vigorous massage and of more copious enemata brought temperature and pulse to still lower register; consciousness, which had been intermittent, fully returned; the swelling in the arm was reduced; and pain had abated. In a week the young man was able to lie at full length, and the swelling, excepting in the ankles was scarcely perceptible. Before this, natural sleep had returned, while temperature and pulse were but slightly above normal. During this interval two enemas daily had been administered, and masses of feces more or less hardened had been removed on each occasion. Sponge baths twice each day had also aided in relieving discomfort while assisting elimination, and at the end of the first week of fasting tub-baths were begun.

The fast was broken on the eleventh day with a small amount of tomato broth fed morning and night, the supply being increased as the patient showed increasing ability to digest his food. Five weeks from the beginning of treatment the youth was enjoying a daily walk of several miles, and thereafter, adhering strictly to the dietetic regimen prescribed, he rapidly developed to a condition of normal health and eventually to a robust physique.

The second case, a man sixty-one years of age, was stricken with paralysis of the entire right side, and, receiving no help from medicine, he determined upon an absolute fast. The preparatory period covered but ten days, a time too short to permit of wholly satisfactory approach to total abstinence, but nevertheless at its completion a fast of forty days, which proved eminently successful in outcome, was undertaken. Paralysis of this nature, known as hemiplegia, is usually caused directly by hemorrhage in some portion of brain tissue. For its relief but one course can be followed—to permit natural processes to absorb the formed blood clot, thus removing inflammation and pressure, releasing nerve force, and allowing connective tissue again to form by natural processes of healing. Constant ingestion of food in the circumstances serves to aggravate and to prolong recovery, since to facilitate the process of absorption the blood should be relieved as rapidly as possible of the burden of waste it has been carrying, waste that in all probability was directly the cause of the brain hemorrhage. The fast by compelling the dominance of elimination at once reduces the density of the blood through removal of circulating refuse, and gives the natural assistance necessary for the disposal of obstructions to the passage of nerve force through nerve channels—thus restoring sensation and motion the loss of which constitutes paralysis.

The patient in question weighed at the time of his apoplectic seizure 228 pounds. Each day of abstinence showed loss in weight, and at the end of the fast the latter was reduced to 174 pounds. Bile in abundance was discharged with the enemas, and at intervals vomiting of the same fluid occurred. The fast was broken with grape-juice and orange-juice, but after a few days more solid food was taken. It is well to quote from a personal letter from the patient, reading as follows:—

"I was totally incapacitated from actual manual labor of any kind before my fast, and I lived in dread of a second stroke, with a strange, unnatural depression evident upon slight over-exertion. Great drowsiness affected me, and on occasions I would sleep thirty to thirty-six hours, almost without intermission. My mentality was impaired, my eyesight defective, and my speech impeded. My right hand and arm were clumsy and weak, and at this stage all ordinary human aid seemed powerless.

"I began the fast, and contrary to my expectations, I had no hunger from the third day to the fortieth. To affirm that there was no inconvenience, however, would be untrue, for by every avenue of elimination most offensive impurities were thrown off, and at times these could not have been borne had the object been lost sight of. My weight before I undertook the fast was 228 pounds, and the girth of my abdomen, 45 inches. After I had completed the total abstinence period,

I weighed 174 pounds, and measured in girth 38-½ inches. I am cured of my paralysis; my mentality is clear and normal; my entire digestive system is apparently perfect; my vision is better than for years; my hand and arm are strong; I have no dread of a second stroke; I have no sleepy spells; I feel lighter all over; and, when weary, I am quite refreshed and ready for further exertion after a short rest."

A case of the disease symptom known as chorea occurring in a woman twenty-eight years of age next offers itself for description. Preparation was undergone for several weeks and a fast of twenty-two days resulted in the return of hunger with complete restoration to health. The medical history of this case showed obstinate constipation for twenty years; and there were nervous tendencies that had been persistently present in aggravated form. Medical advice and direction had been constantly followed since birth, yet, when first seen, the muscles controlling and forming legs, hands, arms, and face were in constant action, and no effort of the will could command them. During the first week of the fast, improvement in the latter respect appeared, so much so that the young woman was able to walk without any evidence of extraordinary lack of coordination, and by the fourteenth day all muscular signs of nervousness had completely disappeared.

No unusual symptoms developed in this case. The enemas brought away solid matter in decreasing amount until the seventeenth day, and thereafter but a small quantity of bilious fluid. Body manipulation and the baths were daily resorted to, and the loss in weight was not remarkable. There were almost no unpleasant symptoms, and this was of the absence of structural organic defect, and because the patient had always led an outdoor life and possessed an equable disposition. After a time devoted to a dietetic regimen and judicious exercises, the case was discharged as restored to health and with no traces of her former nervous disorder. An added benefit was discovered in that, although there had been decided impairment of sight, myopic in character, the patient was able to dispense with lenses six weeks after the beginning of the fast.

The distressing affliction, epilepsy, is a disease symptom that may be traced to the source of all functional disorder, the digestive machinery.

The case of a young woman, twenty-nine years of age, will demonstrate the effect of the fast and its adjuncts upon this characteristic of disease. Before entering the fast, the patient had tentatively followed a dietetic regimen, and had noted decided improvement in general health, but there was no cessation of the attacks peculiar to the symptom named. Medical attendance had been continuous for years, but no improvement had resulted; rather the reverse, for the epileptic seizures had increased in number and severity as time went by. Before the fast the attacks were recurring at intervals of two weeks, and the latest seizure had happened but three days before the fast began. Food was denied for fifty-six days, and, from the moment of the inception of the method to the present writing not a convulsion has occurred, nor has there been a semblance of attack, while in general health the patient has been better than at any time of her life.

The fast in this instance is to be noted in several minor ways, one of which is that on each of the fifty-six days the patient walked a distance of at least two miles; another, that on the fortieth day of abstinence a mass of dead intestinal worms passed from the bowels in the enema. Improvement was constant from the first, but, after the evacuation of these parasites, it increased rapidly, and natural hunger asserted itself on the fifty-fifth day. The loss in weight was consistently normal, averaging about three-quarters of a pound for each day of the fasting period.

The medical history of the next subject, a woman forty-five years old, tells of continuous treatment for thirty years for the disease symptom known as psoriasis in its diffuse form. At the time that the patient sought natural means of assistance the inflamed, bleeding surfaces characteristic of the symptom covered at least one-third of the skin of the body, and they were not confined to any particular locality, appearing indiscriminately upon trunk, arms, and legs, but the hands, face, and feet were not affected. The sores were exuding bloody serum, and there was intolerable itching, so much so that in order to exist in any condition approaching comfort, local application of mercurial preparations had long been resorted to, to relieve both the pain and the inconvenience. These of course were only temporary in effect, and the major symptoms returned shortly, more angry and more obstinate.

The general health of the patient apart from the distressing symptom described was excellent, strange to say. And to this a strong constitution and robust physique in large part contributed. Perhaps, as is at times assumed, the channel taken by nature to rid the body of toxic matter, if sufficiently extensive, precluded the development of other and differing symptoms of disease. This has been held to have been proved in instances of syphilitic infection, which in the majority of cases seems to grant immunity from minor though equally infectious disease, the latter being subordinated to the dominant blood taint.

When first under observation the patient weighed 172 pounds, and her habits were those of a woman in comfortable circumstances with the idea ingrained that three and even four generous daily meals were necessary for the conservation of health and strength. She was, however, disheartened and discouraged because of the almost unbearable distress occasioned by the state of her body, and, as a last resort only, she consented to undergo a fast.

After three weeks of preparation, abstinence from food succeeded and continued without interruption for seventy-five days. At no time during this period was anything excepting water ingested, and at no time was the patient unable to cover on foot the distance from her home to the office of her physician. Once this subject had grasped the philosophy of the method and had experienced the progressive improvement that marked her case, an excellent physical organization and a determined will made her more than equal to the attainment of the object in view, and, as a consequence, she was easy to treat.

The fast was typical and was remarkable in nothing save its length, a phenomenon due again to the extreme resistance which is always discovered in the normally functioning body. Loss in weight not unusual, and at the end of the fast a diminution in this respect of but 32 pounds was noted, the patient then tipping the scales at 140. Until the twentieth day, there was in evidence slightly lowered temperature and pulse, with some chilliness, but, while pulse and temperature remained below register in the early stages of abstinence, by the sixth week normal had been reached. The enemas contained solid feces until about one-third of the fasting period had elapsed, and thereafter, until the last week without food, large amounts of yellowish-white mucus formed part of the discharge. This catarrhal refuse eliminated thus from the intestines indicated that the eliminative function had again been established through normal channels. In fact, a significant feature connected with any symptom of disease of the character expressed in this subject is the failure of function through normal avenues other than the skin to perform, the surface of the body suffering from overwork and disease in consequence.

It was not until the fourth week that visible improvement in exudation from the open sores became noticeable in respect to granulation, although the exudation had begun to diminish during the third week and at this time also the itching had greatly subsided. As healing of the sores progressed, the unpleasant minor symptoms disappeared, healthy skin soon forming in patches that increased in size and gradually covered the denuded spaces.

After breaking the fast, general health continued excellent, and the sole remaining signs of the psoriasis were the scarred edges surrounding areas latest to heal. Even these in time vanished, and no trace, excepting slight discoloration, the result of previous mercurial treatment, was left as a reminder of the hideous and distressful malady of previous years.

While the patient during the first few days of the fast felt some trepidation as to its efficacy and its outcome, after improvement of the condition appeared, its psychological effect was such that her determination to carry on to the return of hunger became fixed. Again it is to be noted that fear enters and disaster results while fasting a functional case only when the method is incorrectly conducted. This case is a supreme example demonstrating the truth that, in the absence of organic disease, there is no danger whatever in abstaining from food until nature asserts by the return of hunger that systemic purification is completed.

Another case presents itself—that of a woman thirty-four years old, partially paralyzed and suffering from general functional disease. In this patient two of the dorsal vertebrae had been displaced in early life in such manner as to compress the spinal cord, thus causing paralysis of the lower trunk and legs. In the absence of any history of accident the only tenable theory of causation of this condition is that of lack of development of the muscles supporting the spine in the dorsal region, this in turn due to faulty nutrition in youth. In all her life this woman had never known a moment of comparative health, and intermittently in earlier day's severe fevers with inflammatory intestinal symptoms had occurred, eventually creating contractions in the colon, a condition that caused constipation and consequent septicemia. When first examined, the case had been bedridden for one year, and it was evident that by reason of the very evident ankylosis existing in the displaced vertebrae referred to there was small hope of correcting the paralysis noted. The symptom that impelled the employment of means other than medicine for relief in this case was an ominous congestive chill from which the woman with difficulty rallied. The fast was entered and carried to what may be regarded as a successful end after fifty-eight days of abstinence.

The medical history of this case showed an inherited tendency towards scrofula or constitutional tuberculosis, and there had been manifested at intervals offensive running sores, the thumb and index finger of the left hand having been amputated some years previous because of a non-healing scrofulous abscess. All of the ulcers that had appeared had, without exception, been diagnosed by attending physicians as tubercular in character and had been treated from the medical viewpoint accordingly.

Two days after the beginning of the fast, an abscess broke through the surface of the skin at the base of the spine immediately over the sacrum. The discharge from this sore was most profuse and offensive, and the area affected spread until it was at least three inches in diameter, with depth such that within ten days after the skin had broken the periosteum of the sacrum was exposed. For a week hot fomentation were continuously applied, and gangrenous tissue in process of formation was cauterized by carefully focusing the rays of the sun upon the ulcer with a large reading glass. By the tenth day the discharge ceased being offensive and shortly thereafter healthy granulation or healing began. When the fast was at an end, the sole evidence of the existence of this sore was a circular spot of slightly reddish normal skin of which a subjacent cushion of soft and healthy tissue showed that natural work of repair had proceeded despite total abstinence from food. This is undoubtedly the point of greatest interest and import to be noted in the treatment and progress of the case, for it is to be remembered that the blood of this woman had in all probability been tainted from birth, and that it had been poisoned and repoisoned for years by continuous addition to accumulated toxic substances. Elimination of body waste had never been successfully accomplished in this patient, but once it could proceed undisturbed in function, nature was able not only to cast out existing impurity, but also to repair diseased tissue by selecting healthy pabulum from the store of nutriment husbanded within.

The discharges resulting from copious daily enemas were noticeable for their exceeding foulness, and for excessive amounts of dark bilious fluid evacuated until about the thirtieth day of the fast. Loss in weight was not exceptional, totaling, as it did, but 20 pounds. When it is considered that the patient weighed but 85 pounds at the beginning of the fast, it is seen that, proportionally speaking, this loss conforms with results tabulated later in the text.

Dates are also of interest in this case, which was under treatment during the winter of 1907-8. The woman died of pneumonia early in 1923. In the interim of full fifteen years, she was able to get about in a wheeled chair, was in good general health, and conducted a business of her own, the only inconvenience she suffered being that incident to her incurable paralysis.

Another instance is that of a woman twenty-eight years old in whom poor nutrition and what is called a bilious temperament occasioned a condition of disease that was expressed in periodical headaches and in melancholia with a tendency toward mania. But for the care and devotion of an older sister, the patient, long before coming under observation, would have been placed in an institution for the insane. In fact, it was because the physician last consulted had recommended that she be restrained that her relatives in despair resorted to the fast.

Examination discovered a pulse continually at 128 or thereabouts with temperature varying from above to below normal by several degrees. Diet had consisted largely of meat and its extracts, this being at once changed to vegetable broths. Daily enemas were thoroughly administered and at first hot towel packs were used upon the spine in order to control circulation and to steady the fluctuating pulse, but these were discontinued shortly as heart action made constant improvement from the beginning of treatment. Dark, foul-smelling discharges that did not cease until the latter portion of the fast formed the bulk of the liquid in the return from the enemas.

This patient also showed extraordinary vigor and vitality throughout a period of forty-two days of abstinence from food, and she daily walked a distance of several miles, underwent manipulative treatment, and returned to her home without undue fatigue. Towards the end of the fast she was able and desirous of increasing the amount of exercise, and her mental condition exhibited improvement from the inception of the work. On the thirtieth day of the fast and thereafter the young woman performed her portion of the housework well and cheerfully. Hunger returned on the forty-first day, and the fast was broken at the end of the forty-second. Two weeks later the sisters sailed for their home abroad, and letters written by the patient since their arrival show a mind in every respect rational.

Tuberculosis of the lungs is a symptom of disease that needs to be uncovered and treated in its early stages if recovery is to be hoped for, and the case of a woman thirty-two years old is cited to illustrate the treatment of a consumptive, the outcome of whose case proved a cure. This patient abstained from food for twenty-four days, but preparation, the fast, and the period of dieting after the latter was concluded, covered full six months. When first under observation, the sputum contained the bacilli typical of the symptom; both lungs were affected; the characteristic cough, high temperature and pulse, were present; in fact, the case displayed all of the signs that distinguish the symptom. The fast was begun after usual preparatory diet, and was continued as noted for twenty-four days, during which no unfavorable symptoms occurred. However, from the latter part of the preparatory period there was excessive discharge of sputum, but during the fast this showed daily diminution in amount, and there was also pronounced decrease in the number of bacilli at the several periodical examinations made. The enemas were charged with bilious products and old feces, these toxic disturbers disappearing only during the last week of abstinence. Fever had vanished as had also the cough by the fourteenth day, and, when the sputum was examined on the twenty-second day of fasting there were no traces of bacilli tuberculosis.

To anticipate successful issue, the treatment of tuberculosis of the lungs should be undertaken before the stage of excessive structural break-down of lung tissue has been reached. If the treatment outlined is begun at this time a cure is altogether probable. Otherwise, the case classes itself with that of advanced organic disease, which, in the light of previous discussion, bars remedy.

Medical diagnosis of the next instance, a man thirty-eight years old, pronounced it a case of valvular heart disease, and medical prognosis gave no hope of recovery. There was severe pain in the regions of the heart, the stomach, and the liver, and at times in the abdomen. Heart-beats were most irregular; and, in view of the very apparent seriousness of the condition, a fast was begun without preparation. Large amounts of dark bilious fluid came away with every enema, and excruciating pain and nervous excitement were experienced until the twentieth fasting day when at least a teacupful of gall-stones was evacuated. Great relief followed, but gall-stones singly and in small numbers were passed with the excreta until the thirtieth day of abstinence. The fast was broken on its thirty-fifth day, when the weight of the patient was 174 pounds, this showing a reduction of 20 pounds within the period given. In the early part of this fast there were slight sub-normal temperature and fasters' chilliness, but temperature and heartbeat as well reached normal by the twentieth day. Before this the pulse had been at times above, at times below register, according to the degree of activity of circulating poison. After breaking the fast all functions became and continued normal; weight was gradually gained and soon reached 185 pounds; and from the completion of treatment general health was excellent.

An interesting addendum to this case is found in its later history. The patient, after strictly adhering to the rules prescribed as to diet, exercise, and general care of the body for at least a year and a half after his restoration to health, lapsed and fell into laxness in eating and in drinking, with the result that, two years subsequent to the crisis already related, an abscess formed upon the fioor of the stomach, and the case again came under observation and treatment, undergoing this time a fast of forty-five days. The man suffered great pain until the ulcer discharged, which occurred about ten days after the fast began, and was evidenced by the passage of blood and pus from the bowels. The patient hovered between life and death for several weeks, but absence of food prevented irritation of the ulcer, which rapidly healed, and, since hunger was in evidence, the fast was broken on the forty-sixth day.

It is the fixed opinion of the author that in no instances is the medical theory of "feeding to keep up strength" so palpably in error, as in cases of the kind just cited. Whether the ulcer is located in the stomach, in the duodenum, or in any other portion of the alimentary tract, non-irritation is a first essential to healing, and non-irritation may be had in the alimentary tract only through the omission of the ingestion of food. And, more, while it is true that food is never essential in disease, the application of the method outlined herein to a condition such as was exhibited in the second siege of illness undergone by the ease just noted is so plain in exposition and so beautifully reasonable and convincing in argument that no unbiased mind should read this description without being satisfied of its truth and in consequence of the efficacy of the method itself.

A short description of a fast for chronic digestive disturbance is presented in the following case, that of a man of forty-five years of age. The fast itself covered a period of forty-nine days, and from its beginning until the forty-fifth day the patient was confined to his bed. This is a striking example of the extreme toxemia that sometimes occurs during fasting when the organs of elimination are called upon to cope with an accumulation of waste that taxes them to the utmost Because this material is liquefied in form, both in consequence of the body secretions and of the water of the enemas, it is more easily absorbed from the walls of the intestines, and in this instance, the weakness in evidence was directly occasioned by this sort of self-poisoning. But the condition gradually improved as the eliminative organs became equal to their tasks, and on the forty-fifth day, hunger returned and with it strength. The fast was broken on the morning of the fiftieth day and afterwards the patient walked several miles on the city pavements with but little fatigue. There were no unusual symptoms other than the toxemia mentioned, and from the breaking of the fast, improvement was constant and permanent.

In another instance the fast was undertaken by a

woman forty-one years old for the purpose of correcting heart irregularity caused by functional disease and obesity. The patient who was under height weighed 200 pounds, and she gave no medical history excepting that some years previous she had been operated upon for chronic inflammation of the fallopian tubes. The fast proper was somewhat lengthy, covering sixty-three days and again it is to be noted that the patient was at all times during abstinence able to attend to her home duties and to make on foot the daily trip to the office of her physician. There was but little fasters' chilliness, and there were no unusual symptoms, excepting that, about the period included between the thirtieth and fortieth days, a gain in weight of from one to two pounds daily occurred, but at the end of this interval gradual decrease in weight again began and continued to the end of the fast, when weight was reduced to 140 pounds. In the meanwhile heart irregularity had disappeared, and by careful attention to her dietary, the patient has succeeded in having no return of the obese symptoms, while general health has been consistently excellent.

Medical diagnosis of the next case classified the symptom as cancer of the stomach. The patient, a man forty years old, was really suffering from an ulcerated condition of the upper portion of the intestinal tract, and he underwent a fast of fifty days in which no marked peculiarities developed. Weight was reduced from 145 pounds to 105 pounds, and the subsequent gain both in weight and in strength was typical. In two months after breaking the fast the patient balanced the scales at 175 pounds.

A young man of twenty-three offers a case of the insanity of syphilis of the type known in medicine as meningitis. In this subject the blood taint was acquired by contact, and, when observed and first under treatment the case was in what is known as the secondary stage of infection. The state of the patient was such that he had but little control over his faculties, both mental and physical. He would answer questions in a slow, drawling, sleepy manner with but small evidence of sanity in his replies unless shocked in some way. He was shameless in response to the calls of nature and showed abnormal erotic tendencies. Weight when treatment began was 150 pounds. After low diet and an absolute fast of twenty-eight days, the time of dieting and of the fast occupying three months, weight was reduced to 110 pounds. From the inception of the fast improvement was continuous, and this applies both to the physical symptoms of the disease and to the mental state of the subject. At the completion of total abstinence there was no evidence of insanity, and at present writing, ten full years from the treatment of the case, no signs of blood taint are in any manner apparent.

A young man, nineteen years old, who had been led into habits of body and of thought detrimental to normal development, became, as a result, a victim of the symptom of disease known as epilepsy. For five years he had suffered from the convulsions characteristic of the malady, recurrent at intervals of from one to two weeks. Medicine had exhausted its resources in this case, which was but another of the "last resort" kind, yet after a short while, the patient and his family were responsive to the results of treatment and thereafter were enthusiastic in carrying out its details. For five months a regimen of restricted diet and of fasting was pursued. The time of total abstinence from food intermittently included in this period was sixty days. All general unfavorable symptoms gradually subsided, and the recurrence of the epileptic seizures became reduced in number to such degree that, at the end of the second short fast, four weeks had intervened between attacks; and, when feeding was permanently resumed, no further seizures were apprehended, nor did they occur. Before disease was fully eradicated the weight of the patient was reduced from 140 pounds to 105 pounds. Increase after the fast took place and at the end of the rebuilding period the young man weighed 148 pounds.

A woman, thirty-six years of age, at the end of the third month of pregnancy developed severe symptoms of cholemia, a condition of the liver in which its functions of conversion and elimination are arrested. Vomiting of dark green bilious fluid took place, and the patient was in a state verging upon coma. Immediate action was demanded, and food was at once omitted, while copious enemas were administered twice daily for the time being. The latter brought away dark and foul discharges which continued with no apparent improvement until the seventeenth day of abstinence.

On the fifteenth, sixteenth, and seventeenth days the patient lay in a semi-conscious state, but she revived on the morning of the eighteenth day, when there was a decidedly favorable change in the character of the bowel passages. Rapid return to consciousness occurred, and increased strength with no unfavorable symptoms marked all succeeding days until the twenty-second, when the fast was broken with fruit juices, and thereafter convalescence proceeded without interruption.

The loss in weight in this case was 22 pounds. Temperature and pulse were continually above individual normal until the latter part of the fast, the former ranging between 99 and 102, and the latter from 80 to 110, although a decided drop in both was always observed after the administration of an enema. No return of nausea occurred after breaking the fast, and thereafter the general health of the patient was excellent. At term an eight-pound child was easily delivered, perfect in development and vigorous in health.

On the fifteenth day of this fast, while the patient was lying in partial coma, as described above, a consultation was held with a former medical associate. The latter advocated, as the only means of saving the life of the mother, the immediate abortion of the fetus, and the abandonment of the fast. His opinion was, however, overruled, and the result of the case justified the stand then taken, for as the attending physician at confinement, five months later, he freely expressed his surprise at the state of health of the mother, the ease with which delivery was had, and the remarkable vitality of the infant, and he acknowledged his error in judgment with a complete reversal of his condemnation of the treatment the patient had undergone.

A case analogous to the one just cited is that of a woman of twenty-seven, wife of a physician.

She was between three and four months pregnant, and was suffering severe pain in the region of the uterus and in that of the stomach. The uterus was discovered to be displaced, and by manipulation and the use of tampons it was put into normal position. Nausea with vomiting was constantly distressing the patient when the case was presented, and an immediate absolute fast was decided upon. However, it was thought best that a preparatory period be observed, and for twelve days the patient subsisted upon liquid diet, after which the fast was begun and continued for thirty days. No unusual symptoms arose during this time, and constant general and specific improvement was noted from the beginning. Nausea decreased with progress and vanished about the twentieth day with no recurrence thereafter. Pulse and temperature were slightly below normal until after eating had been resumed. Preparation for the fast was made upon strained vegetable broths and it was broken upon the same dietary. Solid food was resumed twelve days after the completion of abstinence. At term the patient was delivered of a babe weighing seven pounds, as physically perfect and as healthy a specimen as that described in the previous case. The loss of weight in this instance was an even thirty pounds.

It is to be remarked that the children of these two mothers are not only physically excellent examples, but are also mentally intelligent to a marked degree. These gratifying characteristics are to be attributed in great part to the purification of body undergone by the pregnant women at a stage of gestation early enough to provide for tissue structure in the forming fetal bodies unvitiated by disease in the systems of the mothers.

The statement descriptive of the following case is given in the language of the father of the patient:

"During several weeks prior to his sixth birthday, our oldest boy had complained of sore throat and general lassitude. This finally developed into an acute tonsilitis. On the third or fourth day he complained of pain in both knees, and by evening these joints were swollen and red, and the pain had become so intense that the weight of the bedclothes was unbearable. The physician whom we called—one of the regular school—promptly diagnosed the case as one of inflammatory rheumatism. He advised the use of hot applications to subdue the pain, and insisted on putting the left knee, which was the worse, in a splint so that it could not be moved. On his second or third visit he discovered mitral regurgitation, that common and ominous symptom, showing that the systemic poisoning had affected the valves of the heart. His prognosis was most unfavorable. He said that the acute stage would last probably six weeks, and that it would leave the patient with organic heart trouble.

"At this point we decided to resort to a method

in which we had long believed, but which we had failed to try at the outset of this sickness because we had not realized the seriousness of the case. We discharged the physician and began the treatment described herein under the direction of the author. She took off the splint and gave both knees a careful but thorough rubbing. They had been apparently too sensitive to touch before this, but by the time she had finished the massage, the child said that they felt better. She told us not to bother about his heart or anything else in the line of symptoms, but to stop feeding him, to give him daily baths, enemas, and manipulations—and to watch nature do the rest.

"The pain kept up at intervals, intervals that grew steadily longer, however, for two days, and then it ceased entirely. Before the end of the week, the patient was able to be taken down town on a street car for manipulative treatment. His fast lasted twelve days.

"Later in the summer he had a recurrence of old eye trouble, one resulting from an impure condition of the blood. He had been treated the summer before for this trouble, which had lasted several months. This time we at once began another fast, which continued for twenty-two days. At its end he stripped the bandage off: his eyes one evening and looked at us and we knew that the thing was conquered. During a few of the twenty-two days he had a little orange juice, and at all times he had all the water that he desired. A daily bath and rub were given with a copious enema each morning and evening.

"At the time of writing, two years from the date of the last fast, there has been no recurrence of either the throat trouble, rheumatism, or eye trouble, and a regular physician, a friend of the family, who examined the boy a few months ago, pronounced his heart perfect."

The next case is that of a cancer located on the right eyelid of a man sixty-two years old. This malignant sore had been in evidence for twelve years and the patient had been operated upon for its removal twice in this period. Its third appearance was made in virulent form and consultation with a medical specialist resulted in renewed recommendation of the knife, to which this time the patient refused to submit. He began preparation for a fast which lasted forty-five days, at the expiration of which all that remained of the suppurating sore was a reddish scar of its former seat. Four years later his personal report of the case shows no symptom of recurrence upon eyelid or elsewhere, and an excellent state of general health.

The eradication of this symptom of extreme blood impurity by means of the fast fixes the value of the method in forms of disease that are supposedly incurable. It bears out the contention that disease is one with cure, that cure lies in the application of the single method of nature, elimination, which is one with purification. Cancer is but a symptom of general disease, and it may be eradicated when its ravages have not involved an organ to the degree of rendering it incapable of function.

A cancer, a tumor, are evidences of the economy of

nature in gathering her forces of relief at a single point. This single point, the symptom, is ordinarily plainly apparent. Medicine seeks to "drive it in"; surgery to "cut it out"; and neither, when applied, succeeds in removing the cause. Even though the actual growth and its nearby ramifications are extirpated by means of the knife, nature is still impelled to rid the body of its circulating impurity by the construction of destructive cells, and only blood purification can accomplish a cure.

The next subject, a woman twenty-seven years old, suffered constantly from pain, more or less acute, in the left costar region, near the cardiac orifice of the stomach. She had severe headaches, coupled with nausea and vomiting of bile. Medical diagnosis varied with each physician consulted, and the young woman was treated within a period of several years for ailments ranging from ulceration of the stomach to appendicitis. In the course of her search for health she had made visits to famed sanatoria, but her condition steadily grew worse, and, because of it, she was rapidly verging upon melancholia. Hearing of the fast, she was at first interested, then hopeful, and on her own initiative she undertook short periods of abstinence with decided relief. The case was one that, when first observed, showed signs of obstinate intestinal obstruction, which might or might not prove to be a morbid growth, and caution was essential even during the preparatory work. But it was finally determined that a soup and salad regimen be followed, and the dietary indicated was continued for four months with gradual but not permanent relief. However, at the end of this time an attempt was made to change to solid food, when the system at once strongly rebelled, and the patient was actually forced into total abstinence. She fasted forty-three days.

During the early portion of the fast there were headaches and vomiting of greenish bile and mucus, and these distressing symptoms were present until the thirtieth day, when the patient was compelled to take to her bed. The stomach had at all times resisted ingestion even of water, and in order to facilitate the discharge of bile and to reduce nausea, natural stomach-lavage was daily performed. This was done by having the patient drink warm water in quantity and then induce vomiting. Enemas and baths were administered in the usual number and manner. Body manipulation, with especial attention directed to the region under the left lower ribs, was carefully carried out, for by this time it had become obvious that the intestinal obstruction was caused by fecal impaction. On the forty-third day of the fast a broken-up mass of hardened fecal matter was passed with the enema. Extreme relief followed, and the fast was at once discontinued with gratifying results, the stomach accepting the broths, and normal digestion taking place. The feces passed were in the form of balls, black in color and extremely hard in character. This accumulation had been the cause of the symptoms described, all of them signs of exaggerated toxemia. Rapid recuperation ensued.

For a year after the experience related the patient followed a strict dietary, and during this time she underwent a total of forty-five days of short periods of fasting. Her diet consisted in the main of raw tomatoes, hot tomato broth, and salads. At present writing, more than three years from the beginning of the first fast, the young woman is in excellent health.

This case may be considered as perhaps the most aggravated instance of toxemia in the entire history of practice recorded herein. Life was saved only because the patient was constantly under observation, day and night, and distressing and dangerous symptoms were dealt with, as they developed, promptly and skillfully. The case also exemplifies the contention of the writer that at no time, even when acute crises occur, are special, fanciful auxiliaries necessary to combat conditions. Enemas, baths, body manipulation—all natural accessories—invariably prove fully equal to the task.

Without citing individual instances, attention is here directed to the ease with which certain symptoms, to which in recent years the surgical branch of medicine has devoted much time and energy, yield to the fast and its accessories. The vermiform appendix in the human body is a slender blind sac, opening from the cecal portion of the large intestine. It is on an average from three to six inches in length, and of a caliber of that of a lead pencil. It is found in man and in some of the lower animals, and in a few of the latter it is large and performs a digestive function. In the human body its use seems to be more of a question of professional argument than one of determination, but it is quite probable that its function is that of stimulating peristalsis either through the secretion of a lubricant or by muscular contraction.

Inflammation of the vermiform appendix constitutes true appendicitis. In the medical world appearance of this symptom demands immediate operation with removal of the offending organ. Observation of numbers of alleged cases of appendicitis leads to the belief that an inflamed appendix is a symptom of disease most rare in occurrence. Because the function of this organ has not been satisfactorily determined by science, and because its absence from the body seemingly creates no lack of harmony among other essential parts of the organism, extirpation has become the rule. And there has been exercised in this connection a great deal of snap judgment in diagnosis. Gas formed in the cecum, gall stones in the gall sac, inflammation of the right ovary and of the bowel in the ileo-cecal region, all have been mistaken for an appendix inflamed, and have occasioned operations unnecessary in the extreme with serious and perhaps fatal results.

In the treatment of any intestinal inflammation, appendicitis included, no assistance is needed other than that which complete rest of the digestive tract and constant use of the enema afford. When no complications exist, the fast causes inflammation to subside, pain to cease, and fever to be reduced, by, at the most, the third day of abstinence, and the sole necessity for continuing the fast is found in seeking best and lasting results.

Fasters' chilliness has been referred to a number of times, and it is as well to say here that body temperature when this sensation is in evidence is always more or less below normal in register. This feeling of chill may be attributed partly to the absence of food stimulation, but it is largely due to permeation of the circulation by bilious products that, in the circumstances, create, not fever, but a nervous reaction that causes muscular and skin contraction with an appreciable drop in body heat and probable lowered heart beat. It is to be recognized that so-called normal pulse and normal temperature terms that are relative, and that the limits placed upon them as standard vary in different persons, as do physical peculiarities. In some of the cases described and in others not mentioned, temperature and pulse remained below register during a portion of the fasting period, but as systemic cleansing progressed, average individual normal was gradually restored. When fasters' chilliness occurs, the hot therapeutic bath must frequently be resorted to in order that muscular relaxation may occur, thus permitting the temporarily inhibited eliminative function of the skin to be restored.

Organic rest and systemic purification, resulting from the employment of the fast and its auxiliary eliminative agencies, form the basis of the method outlined in the text. The fast, than which no greater eliminative agent is known, is the fundamental of treatment, but additional natural therapeutic means that may in any manner assist in attaining results are never to be ignored, and these material auxiliaries are in most senses foreign to the domain of medicine. Manipulation of the body, specific and general, intelligently applied, proves of greatest worth during a fast and thereafter. Adjustment of the spinal column has its own especial place as a valuable accessory of treatment. And each of these therapeutic measures, with others that have been described, while not to be thought of as a panacea, is yet to be considered as an important adjunct in the natural treatment of disease.

Caution and Counsel

6

Competent Guidance is Required for Protracted Fasts: Short Fasts: Corrective Dietary

Much though it is to be desired by those who know the inestimable benefits to be derived from a fast that is scientifically conducted, there is but small hope that this natural means of bodily purification, of disease eradication, will ever prove a popular method of health restoration. Self-denial and self-control are two virtues that the average mortal is content to relegate to the side-lines in the game of life. Or, if he be not content so to do, it is easy to shift responsibility to those whose profession it is to prescribe a remedy the purpose of which is to suppress the manifest symptom, to ease present distress or disturbance. The cause of local expression, of the symptom or symptoms, has no place in a philosophy of this character, yet, unless the source of disease is attacked and removed, health is really never his who depends upon symptomatic alleviation. And again, when one is ill, no real self-denial or control is needful to curtail or even entirely to omit food. And, while it is many times accentuated in the text that food withdrawal is the easy, and at once the natural and the scientific measure to be employed whenever illness occurs, since hunger and disease never exist simultaneously in the animal body, few possess courage to apply it.

Now, while in acute or chronic disease there are difficulties to be encountered in prolonged fasting, the results of a "fast to a finish", to the cleansed systemic condition produced by the process of elimination thus engendered, are nevertheless those that thereafter, with proper care of the body, insure continued normal physical existence. And, as above stated, nature constantly indicates abstention from food in disease, but especially does she do so when acute prostrating illness develops, as well as when certain symptoms, become chronic in character, are present.

In more than thirty years of experience with the fast as a therapeutic agency, the writer has discovered that by far the most satisfactory diet upon which to break a fast is one confined to vegetable broths or soups, prepared in such manner as to preserve both vitamin and mineral content, excluding at the same time all but finely comminuted solid matter. Broths thus made, when eaten slowly, are fully insalivated, easily digested, and their food material is absorbed and assimilated without difficulty. In casting about for a dietary that would accomplish these ends, much observation and experiment were in order, and in the course of investigation it was determined that where, in functional disease, a fast protracted in length made upon its subject demand for absolute rest, hence precluding attention to daily duty in business or otherwise, a diet restricted to soups similar to those upon which a fast is broken in great degree permitted the function of elimination to preponderate, satisfied stomach craving if present, and did not, excepting in slightest measure, interfere, either psychologically or physiologically, with intake and outgo of vital force.

Naturally when corrective eating is substituted for fasting, the process of bodily purification, of systemic cleansing, is prolonged; but the symptoms produced are in modified form similar to those noted during the progress of an absolute fast continued to its logical end, the return of natural hunger. And the results that accrue, though delayed and not equal to those obtained by a "fast to a finish," are eminently satisfactory.

For many reasons, quite obvious ones too, complete abstention from food in illness occasions in those who are uninformed upon the benefits that follow in its train, and who are ignorant of the physical resources of the human body and of the physiological changes that abstinence occasions, thoughts that are decidedly deterrent. And this though, as is so often iterated herein, no real desire for food exists at the time. The patient himself may be fully cognizant of body resource and of the advantages that follow abstinence, and he may possess the necessary will to impose upon himself the discipline needful for successful issue; but in the usual instance there are relatives and friends, who are not, as is the sufferer, in touch with nature, and here opposition often evolves that in effect annuls the action, if not the inclination. On the other hand, there is this to be said: if the patient has the will and the determination to carry to conclusion an absolute fast, if, *under guidance during its continuance,* he employs the essential eliminative agencies, and, if no serious organic condition is uncovered, as it surely will be if it exists, relief with recovery will occur much more rapidly and satisfactorily than is possible when even the small amount of sustenance contained in the restricted regimen described is ingested.

And this brings us to the purpose of this short chapter, which is intended both as caution and as counsel. No one, unless so acutely ill as to be compelled to do so, should attempt protracted abstinence from food unless competent guidance is available. The "fast to a finish" is not an affair for personal conduct. In it organic disease may be uncovered, and from day to day after the first week or so symptoms may and will develop that need to be dealt with by the expert hand. Without the advice and encouragement of one skilled in the therapy of inanition fear may drive out courage, and then hasty and ill advised attempts to relieve mental and physical distress will surely entail calamitous issue.

But for him to whom the tenets of the text appeal a happy mean exists. In incipient illness, in times of slight physical depression when preventive measures are in order, or when functional disturbance of character more or less severe occurs, then shorter periods of abstention from food may safely and with benefit be personally employed. The omission of food for periods ranging from one to ten days need in the ordinary instance occasion no difficulty nor engender fear. But always the eliminative accessories that are dwelt upon in connection with fasting, absolute or partial, and with restricted diet in illness, are faithfully to be used. Daily colon flushing, daily cleansing baths, and every aid to elimination through every natural channel must accompany and assist the basic procedure.

Alternating with these shorter fasts there should occur intervals of corrective dieting, and the broths already mentioned, prepared to suit individual taste and requirement, will here fit the condition presented. The soups may be varied in ingredients, and one pint is in amount sufficient for one meal. Baths and enemas should he taken as during the fasting stage, but their administration is to be timed so as not to interfere with digestive function. Preferably they should precede the meal, allowing at least an interim of about one hour before ingestion. It may be that in certain cases the system will for a time object to the ingestion of the specially prepared broths. Fruits, however, may be and usually are tolerated, and here a change may be made to a dietary of fruit alone, taking care that but a single sort be eaten at a meal and that this be perfectly ripened.

Children in illness readily respond to the fast, yet, with growing bodies and with undeveloped physical resource, the absolute fast, excepting for periods one or several days in duration, is, unless there is acute disease, here to be inhibited. But always recourse may and should be had to the one-food dietary, either interrupted or continuous, at the same time, as for the adult, plying enemata and cleansing tub baths.

In the list of vegetables that may be utilized for the preparation of broths none can quite take the place of the tomato. This plant occupies a position that lies between the classifications of fruit and vegetable; it contains food elements of every sort in varying proportion, including relative parts of virtually all of the mineral matter needful for systemic maintenance, being especially rich in potassium and sodium; and it carries the three essential vitamins, "A", "B", and "C". Its acid content is one that acts in the nature of a solvent, aiding in the digestion of other foods. Used when thoroughly ripe, in its natural or in its canned state, it satisfies both taste and nutrition, and broth made from it is the ideal form of sustenance for breaking a fast and for use during times of corrective eating, when the latter are interspersed with short fasts. There are subjects by whom a diet of tomato alone may be eaten with benefit for several weeks or longer, excluding the while intervals of total abstinence from food, but always employing the eliminative aids. The onion is also valuable in this respect, and a "tomato fast" or an "onion fast", weeks in duration, may ordinarily be personally conducted with great benefit when the eliminative accompaniments are included in the procedure.

It is explained that for the purposes of the text to fast means to abstain from all food material save water. The latter is to be used at all times for drinking, whether the subject be fasting or dieting—this when thirst demands. But during abstinence drinking increased quantities of water, hot or cold, makes for solvency and assists in replenishing body fluids, and in flushing body organs.

In summation, long experience confirms the conclusion that fasting protracted in length of duration should never be undertaken unless the subject be under competent direction. In usual instances, even though essential accessory detail be faithfully observed, personal conduct may and probably will, for reasons given, lead to disaster. But a series of short fasts, interspersed with intervals of corrective eating, may with safety and with benefit be personally conducted, as may periods of partial abstinence on the one-food plan, the latter liquid in form. It remains to be added that many times, in order to secure best results, the competent director will deem it advisable or essential to make use of the interrupted or of the one-food fast when dealing with temperaments who by nature possess or who develop in disease certain mental or physical idiosyncrasies.

Preparation for the Fast 7

True Hunger Disappears When Disease Approaches: Tapering off to a Complete Fast: The Function of the Liver: Two Plans for Fasting

When disease appears in humankind, it is, as said before, not only a cautionary but a curative process. A disturbing element needs removal; tired and abused organs need rest and repair. Instinctively real food desire, true hunger, disappears; in fact, for some time previous to actual disability, hunger has been absent. Appetite or stimulated demand for sustenance may, however, be in evidence and may remain in evidence even after illness is manifest; but disease and hunger cannot exist at the same time in the human body.

Bodily functions are swift in their adaptability to conditions, and bodily organs accommodate themselves and their labors even to abuse. Consequently, in a system accustomed to continuous excess food supply, nature carries on existence in spite of handicap until accumulation and subsequent decomposition institute disease. Could the subject recognize that prevention of later evil lies entirely in his own hands, the greater portion of physical suffering would be eradicated; but prevention compels personal denial of personal habit and enjoyment; and denial in this respect is the hardest of all virtues to inculcate and to practice.

The simplicity of the application of the fast constitutes one of its principal drawbacks. To a mind convinced on final argument of the efficacy of the method, nothing is easier than to begin the omission of the daily ration, irrespective of the mental and physiological changes that are involved. But food stimulation, always an important factor in disease, asserts the power of habit over the body; and, even though the will of the patient has been brought to understand the futility of dependence upon artificial aids to health, as embodied in medicine and in methods akin to it, general knowledge is lacking concerning the proper means to pursue in order to overcome habit and to meet the physiological changes that ensue when food is denied the body for the purpose of prevention or of cure of disease.

The cultivation of a habit is a slow and insidious process, and so, in lesser degree perhaps, is its destruction. Abruptly to cease an action, normal or abnormal, habitually connected with bodily function, causes both physical and mental disturbance. Witness, for instance, the attempts of a victim of tobacco, alcohol, or morphine to escape from the toils. In the ordinary case will power alone may accomplish the result sought for.

But in the purifying process of the fast abnormal desire is removed, and physical habits of this sort are thus easily conquered.

In many cases the will required to begin a fast is present, and, were this the sole consideration, food might at once be denied. But, because natural physiological change is always gradual in accomplishment, a like approach to cessation of digestion is essential. The ideal manner of effecting the readjustment of organic action, the consequence of lowering to zero the intake of food, is to diminish by degrees the amount ingested, for suddenly to omit food at the inception of a fast sets the stomach clamoring for supply at the hours which habit has fixed, and the results of deprivation are then comparable to those experienced by the toper or the drug victim when drink or narcotic is denied. Nervous reaction is at once apparent and depression follows. Only in acute disease should abrupt entrance be made to the fast, and this solely because at such times nature makes the issue and removes effectively all desire for food.

Daily baths and enemata, natural means for external and internal cleansing of the body and aids to elimination which do not disturb function as do purgatives, mark the commencement of treatment; and these accompaniments, with the omission of the midday meal, embody the first stage of approach to the period of total abstinence from food. Omitting the noon meal and lessening quantity at other meals paves the way; and, in the ordinary instance of functional disease, gradual diminution of food supply should occupy an interim of about ten days or two weeks, after which tomato broth, onion broth, or some similar light fluid food, in limited quantity, may be used, dropping then to lemon juice with honey in hot water taken about three times daily. In fact, half a lemon and a dessert spoon of honey to a pint of hot water may in many instances be given with benefit several times each day during the non-food interval. The slight effort of digestion required for this usually pleasant beverage does not to any degree interfere with the eliminative processes, and in cases where suggestion may be used with profit, it performs this service.

If as sometimes happens the omission of the mid-day meal occasions distress, ripe fruit in small quantity may be eaten at the usual hour. Soups made of vegetables gradually becoming lighter in food value should constitute the morning and evening meals until they are dispensed with, and then it is well to use the lemon and honey as described or the juices of fruit alone for the last few days preceding the fast itself.

In the ordinary patient the omission of the noon meal may cause slight disturbances, such as dizziness, headache, or stomach craving. These are mostly the results of habit change, and usually they disappear within three or four days, when there are commonly no further unpleasant symptoms as the remaining meals are omitted. In the two-meal period elimination of digestive toxins begins to gain over their formation, and, as the patient gradually lowers ingestion, it becomes most evident, from the discharges in the enemata and from the odor that emanates from skin and breath, that the body is undergoing strenuous housecleaning. These phenomena make it apparent that previous continuously overburdened digestive function, with consequent defective nutrition, has filled the entire system with toxic products, and that complete purification, coupled with rest for the organs of digestion and those allied with them is necessary for regaining physical balance. A new foundation is to be constructed as the old is removed, and a change in physiological condition is to be effected by casting from the body the active cause of disease, and by renewing, through cell reconstruction and rest, the functioning ability of those organs that long have been hampered in operation.

At the portal of the circulation of the blood, like a faithful sentry, stands the liver. The function of this organ is to receive digested food after its absorption through the villi, which are short hair-like processes residing on the walls of the intestines, and designed for this purpose. Receiving digested food in this manner, the liver then proceeds to separate it into that which may be used for rebuilding of tissue and that which is waste. Its products are, on the one hand, tissue-nutriment, and, on the other, the peculiar secretion known as bile. Bile, even when normal in character, is essentially a waste product, and, after separation by the liver, it is stored in the gall sac, whence it is discharged into the intestines and utilized in the digestive processes. Nature is loath to cast out any material as useless, and one of the most striking instances in her economy is this utilization of an essentially waste product in the digestive function.

When overworked by overfeeding or other abuse, the liver cannot successfully perform its task of inspection, and the bile retained is carried into the blood current. Surplus of this fluid is also apparent intestinally in these circumstances, and with it the headache, the cold, or a bilious crisis occurs.

The minute cells of the liver have individual work to perform in separating nutritive matter from waste; and, unless care be taken to furnish a food supply correct in proportion and quality, bile is secreted and excreted in quantity greater than the system requires, and is itself absorbed and reabsorbed, with additions from other sources, until congestion results, the circulation is vitiated, and the bowels are filled with bilious toxins poison and repoison indefinitely. All habits having a tendency to cause digestive disturbance, such as the use of tobacco or alcohol, careless eating and overeating, hinder the functioning of the liver. Any interference with its duties prevents the blood from receiving the benefit of its inspection, and an impure product is the consequence. All parts of the body show distressing symptoms of fatigue and exhaustion when the cells of the liver become diseased through intemperate living and ignorance of the specific duty of the organ as a member of the human machine. And this, of course, is true with reference to the functions of any other of the vital parts of the body; but so closely is the work of the liver connected with that of the processes of digestion that detailed description of it and its labors is deemed essential to full understanding of the method discussed herein.

As has been indicated, there are two plans to be followed when the fast is employed as a means for the relief and cure of disease. One of these requires the patient to continue the period of abstinence from food to its logical conclusion, the return of natural hunger. The length of this period depends upon individual physiological peculiarity and organic condition. The other plan makes use of shorter intervals of abstinence, alternating with periods of lowered but corrective diet. What has been written may then be qualified to the degree that, when short fasts of one or two days, or of a week, are undertaken for the relief of slight indisposition or for the prevention of acute disease, no such extended preparation as is described is needful. For the longer fasts, the fasts that cleanse the system to purity, preparation as outlined must be precedent. The short fast and the compulsory fast of acute disease alone may be abruptly begun. However, extended preparation for a fast is to be preferred in all cases where it may be employed. It serves to lessen physiological shock, it curtails the length of the total abstinence period, and in all senses is to be considered as a beneficial process of gradual purification.

8 Symptoms Occurring During Fasting

What Symptoms Mean:

Variety of Symptoms Produced by Elimination

Symptoms of disease are the evidences of abnormal conditions that are present within the body, and they indicate with more or less accuracy the degree of functional or of organic disturbance. In addition they enable the experienced observer to apprehend the point or points of least resistance, the organ or organs that are hampered in the performance of function. In fasting, these signs of disease, during the first days of abstinence, are seen to be exaggerated or increased in severity; but this is a logical consequence of the method as applied, for its purpose is that of elimination of circulating, clogging, poisonous material. The extreme process of elimination in operation at this time fully uncovers the focus of disease, and exaggerates in the very cure itself signs characteristic of morbid conditions in the organs involved, organs whose resistance has been assailed to the point of break-down in function. To the orthodox view this phenomenon at once is suggestive of an increase in the severity of disease alone, since in the commonly accepted opinion the symptom represents a segregated cause. But, rightly regarding disease as arising from a single primary source, the intellect trained in the application of natural means of treatment finds cause for rejoicing rather than for fear. Exaggeration of symptom is apparent because nature has accepted the open road presented, and is proceeding rapidly to effect relief and cure. And it is to be observed that the greater the struggle made at this time, the greater the vital force in reserve.

In any method for the treatment of disease nothing can be done unless nature cooperates. In some methods her means of cure, elimination, triumphs in spite of treatment, and this is nowhere so fully demonstrated as in traditional orthodoxy, which regards the symptom as disease in segregated form. By means of drugs and measures allied, the signs manifested are checked, suppressed, turned into other channels. The fact has been and is ignored that, with cause thus suppressed but still in action, disease is certain of return in aggravated form.

To delay treatment in order that a distinct symptom may develop, thus permitting of accurate symptomatic diagnosis, is evidence of faulty conception both of the character of disease and of its remedy. While waiting, the case is proceeding either to cure or to death. At the first appearance of distress active natural measures are in order, and these are certainly not to be classed with drugs or with any means for the suppression of a localized pathological condition.

For centuries the human race has been educated therapeutically by precept and argument diametrically opposed to truth. For instance, in the orthodox method of handling the sick, if heart action is high, a depressant is administered; if it is low, a stimulant is given. When signs of illness appear upon the skin, attempts are in order, not to remove the inward cause, but to eradicate the outward sign, "to drive it in." In these instances, because of energy consumed in fighting both disease and drug, reaction occurs, and the organs affected are less able to recuperate when the obstructed avenues of vitality are finally cleared sufficiently for function. The latter occurs when nature, as she often does, asserts herself despite the drug. Orthodoxy refuses to admit the unity of disease and cure, and likewise refuses to assist nature in the purifying process of disease. The thought and hope of the physician trained to regard disease from its natural concept is this: that the organs of the body of his patient may prove equal to the work of elimination; and to further this end, he makes use of every natural eliminative aid. In spite of the mildness or the severity of its manifestation, it is only through bodily purification that disease may be cured.

Since the physiological changes involved in the application of fasting for the cure of disease need to be made gradually, as has been related, the ideal method of approach to the period of abstinence is to prepare the system by lessening by degrees the intake of food;

but, whether begun in this manner or without preparation, as is necessary in acute crises, resultant symptoms are in general alike. When the intake of food is stopped, the stomach is naturally emptied and commences its enforced vacation. All energy heretofore applied to the processes of digestion is now directed into eliminative channels, and, with the assistance of a blood current continually growing in purity, inflammation that may be present is allayed, and congestion in veins and glands is relieved. The stomach will from time to time be disturbed by its neighboring organ, the liver which during a fast is solely an organ of elimination, and which then discharges its bilious excretion in large amounts into the alimentary canal It has been stated that this product of the liver is essentially waste, but that, even so, it has its use as a digestive fluid in health. However, when a fast is in progress, bile is profusely poured into the intestines, and it is then to be regarded as naught but poisonous refuse excreted by tissue, and it is at once to be removed from the system lest it be again absorbed into the circulation.

When food is no longer being ingested, the bowels proceed to evacuate their fecal contents, receiving and casting out the waste then deposited in them from blood and the visceral organs; the kidneys, the lungs, and the skin assist in the purifying process; in short, the sewerage system of the body centers its entire energy in supreme effort to overcome toxemia by clearing away internal impurities. The involuntary absorptive functions are, however, still active, and they continue their work, even upon excreted waste; hence, lest poisonous reabsorption occur, the most expeditious means must be employed in order to remove this refuse from the intestinal channel. The blood, following its mission, gathers excrete from cell structure, and supplies what it may for rebuilding purposes. The latter it discovers in that reserve supply of nourishment that is naturally stored in the interstices of tissue. As the process of elimination or purification continues, as refuse diminishes in amount, the density of the blood stream is gradually reduced, and the labor of the heart is thus progressively lightened.

In some diseased conditions the action of the heart is low, in others, it is high. While it is reasonable to expect that the beat of the heart will show lower register when the blood is laden with waste and is dense in quality, after all, physiological temperament determines heart action both normal and abnormal. Disease in some subjects is invariably accompanied with fever and a rapid pulse; in others a sluggish heart with lowered temperature prevails. But whether in disease heart action be high or low, poisonous substances are present in the blood, and these acting upon the nerves that control the heart, the latter may develop irregularities that seem to indicate organic defect, and that are often so diagnosed. But, following the argument of the text, it is obvious that, whatever the symptom, improvement in heart action must necessarily result in a fast when elimination has advanced sufficiently to have removed the major portion of poison circulating in the blood.

No fear need be entertained concerning the ability of the heart to perform its function during a fast, for the organ, as each day goes by has lighter work to do, and it is served with the increasing nerve power of a system that is gradually purifying itself.

As soon as a fast is entered, elimination asserts its predominance. In many instances desire for food is replaced by repugnance, and there is no hunger until the process of purification is completed. The very odor of food, and even the perfume of flowers are to some subjects annoying. In aggravated form this symptom offers the possibility of serious organic deficiency. This statement is not to be taken as conclusive or as a rule, for often in cases in whom bilious excretion predominates, eases whose illness is purely functional in origin, the symptom described occurs. In any event it should be carefully studied and its immediate causes analyzed.

In some instances patients have claimed the sensation of false hunger, of appetite, from the beginning to the end of the fast, but this was due to irritative conditions. There are variations in this sign, more or less to be attributed to the time devoted to the preliminaries, and, when the fast is properly begun and properly continued, neither false hunger nor true hunger is ever in evidence until the end.

Another symptom always present is the thick yellowish-white coat donned by the tongue during abstinence from food. This is in evidence until the impurities of the body are eliminated, and the clearing of the surface of the tongue is one of the positive signals that indicate a complete and successful fast. This coat deposited upon the tongue is perhaps the simplest sign of a foul internal state, and it is also an indication that elimination of impurities is taking place. When food stimulation due to excess supply dominates elimination, the coated tongue, then invariably present, signifies the effort of nature to rid the system of gathering waste. At times during a fast, when the secretions of the body continue to be acid in character, an apparently clean tongue may develop, and in this event strict interpretation of the symptom might lead to the inference that the system is cleansed and is ready again for feeding. The "acid tongue" is easily recognized, for pulse and temperature assist in guidance, while it is altogether probable that additional evidence of its cause will be discovered in the appearance of small ulcers or cankers upon the mucus membrane of the mouth or upon the tongue itself.

Like the tongue, the breath becomes laden with disagreeable evidences of a foul interior, and during the earlier portion of the fasting period, its odor is most offensive. Gradual improvement in this respect is an indicator of the progress of purification which the body is undergoing, and the termination of a successful fast is heralded by an odorless breath.

One of the products of fermentation within the body during disease is known by the name of acetone. There is no doubt that acetone, the result of the decomposition of organic matter, is present in greater or lesser degree in many cases during the fast. It is not at any time necessarily a product of the albumen of food, but is more probably the result of the destruction of that part of the body albumen that has come from the breaking down of tissue cells, waste that, instead of being normally eliminated, is retained with consequent decomposition. In other words, the material that produces acetone has served its purposes as living cell growth. In cases under medical treatment its presence is regarded with dread, and at times when it appears, as it is apt to in anaesthetized subjects under the knife of the surgeon, operations have been abandoned because of the fear of death while the paralysis of the anaesthetic endures. Its appearance in a patient undergoing a fast is an indication of derangement of more than ordinary gravity. In health there is no production of acetone, since discarded cell waste is eliminated before fermentation can occur. Once food is denied and cell refuse is discharged into the channels of evacuation, acetone, when it is present, appears in all the excretions, and its characteristic ether-like odor is most pronounced. In cases like these one of the signs of the beginning of the end of the fast is discovered in the disappearance of acetone from urine, breath, and excrete generally. It is then no longer formed, since the body is again in position to produce normal healthy cell structure balanced by normal elimination of waste.

In disease it is quite usual to observe body odors

that are unpleasant. These are again manifestations of foulness within, manifestations signifying that toxins exist, and that nature is seeking to remove them through every organ of elimination, not the least of which is the skin. One experienced in handling mental disease soon becomes expert in distinguishing the marked odor attached to most lunatics. Even in the milder forms of nervous derangement, such as hysteria, emanation from the body is distinctly changed, so much so that it is frequently noticed by the patient himself. Effluvium, usually disagreeable in character, is present in disease other than that connected with the mental processes and with the nerves—witness, for instance, the distinctive odor of the victim of pulmonary tuberculosis. Because of the predominance of the eliminative function during a fast, the smell of the body is then decidedly more perceptible than is the case in functional disease when food is supplied. So true is this that the presence of a fasting subject can at once be detected by one familiar with the phenomena of the method. The excretions at this time are strongly impregnated with bile, and the peculiar odor that is characteristic of this fluid is most apparent. This results because the entire system has been called into eliminative action, and temporary saturation is the result. The breath is laden with this ill-smelling exhalation until purification is complete, and the skin carries it until the latter point is reached in the progress of the fast.

In cases of acute illness and in what are characterized as bilious temperaments, after the beginning of a fast, annoying symptoms may develop—dizziness on rising suddenly, spots before the eyes, and general malaise and weakness. But these signs are not discovered in all instances and they cannot be established as guides. Some there are who abstain from food for as many as thirty or forty days without disagreeable symptoms other than the offensive and the coated tongue. In these instances vital organs are fully capable of function and are equal to their tasks. On the other hand, there are those in whom all of the signs described are in evidence in varying intensity until nearly the end of the fast. The latter are those who suffer from extreme functional derangement or who possess vital organs that are structurally defective.

To those, who, through high-living and overfeeding, have given the liver work beyond its capability, the experience of the fast is often trying. Bile is cast out in large amounts and floods the intestines to such extent that, often before it can be carried downward, some of it finds its way into the stomach, with nausea and vomiting as sequelae. There is no absolute certainty of the appearance of this sign, but it is usually present in the subjects referred to. In extreme form nausea with vomiting suggests either the presence of an obstruction in the small intestines situated below the opening of the gall duct, or that of organic disease of the liver. If the latter exists, the vomited fluid is ordinarily blackish in color; if the former be the case, the bile vomited is usually yellow or greenish-yellow in tint. In any event the symptom is distressing and it may be more or less serious as to cause, but a number of instances with it intermittently in evidence are noted that progressed to favorable outcome.

The above remarks may be amplified by stating that, for the reason that excessive vomiting of bile during a fast is a symptom that indicates the probability of organic disease of the liver or an obstruction of the intestinal tract, in these cases caution is urged in the employment of the protracted fast. The symptom is not to be regarded as alarming when the fluid raised is yellow or greenish-yellow in hue, nor when nausea occurs at infrequent intervals. But if its color be a vivid green or, as in instances of extreme organic derangement, blackish in tint, the case may be considered as serious in character and of doubtful prognosis. In any event, when nausea is present during a fast, it is far better to rid the stomach of its contents through the mouth than to permit them to remain with the certainty of absorption and toxication. For this purpose drinking of warm water, a quart or so at a time, will ease the act of retching, and at the same time will cleanse the stomach. If difficulty is found in vomiting, titillation of the palate with the end of the index finger will usually suffice to cause the muscular contraction necessary. And this sort of stomach lavage is much more simple in operation and just as efficacious as that by means of a pump. In fact, whenever during a fast there is reason to suppose that the stomach because of inaction has gathered secretion upon its walls, cleansing of the organ in the manner described is in order, and it is always beneficial.

There are patients with livers organically diseased who undergo a fast with no appearance of bilious vomit. Observation in post mortem examination leads to the conclusion that these subjects usually are affected with some form of cirrhosis, and the instances referred to were in body of thin and wiry type. On the other hand, those in whom excessive vomiting occurs during fasting usually are inclined to obesity, and, if organic disease exists and death follows, post mortem examination will in all probability show a liver deteriorated or degenerated in structure.

Bile forced into the stomach may produce through irritation spasmodic contractions of the diaphragm, or hiccoughs. These may also occur because of other stimulation of the diaphragmatic nerve, a frequent happening in cases of functional disturbance of the liver or of the small intestines. When the reason for this annoying symptom is purely functional in character, it may ordinarily be quickly relieved by drinking water or by inducing vomiting; but, if it persists, the case at once assumes gravity in prognosis, for in all probability extreme organic defect has been uncovered. This observation is entitled to additional credence because of several instances in whom persistent hiccoughing occurred shortly before death, and in whom the autopsies revealed organic disease of the upper portion of the small intestine.

In the earlier stages of a fast there will probably be fermentation with consequent formation of gas in the bowels, and this may continue for a few days, depending upon the amount of waste retained, and upon what may be termed the virulence of the bilious excretion deposited in the intestinal tract. The gas formed is often the cause of colicky pains, and is always a source of uncomfortable moments until it is discharged. To this end manipulation of the abdomen and hot water applications upon its surface are of much assistance. By these measures peristalsis is stimulated, and the inflated bowel is reduced by forcing the gas to the rectum, thence to discharge. However, the enema is to be regarded as the greatest ally of the body for the assistance of bowel evacuation, and it should be resorted to in the circumstances related and in all other similar situations.

In all cases in the fast the evacuations from the bowels are much alike. At first old feces more or less abundant in quantity are discovered floating in a brownish fluid that often shades to black. Solid waste is usually present for a number of days, although its amount depends in great measure upon the time devoted to preparation for the total abstinence period. These formed feces offer definite evidence of the truth of the statement that an overloaded colon does not fully evacuate its contents even though daily passages are the rule.

At some point or other in the purifying process there appear in the evacuations stringy masses of white or yellowish mucus. In catarrhal cases these are discovered at the beginning of treatment and they usually continue in evidence until purification of the system is completed. In other subjects mucus commonly does not appear until the fast is well under way, but it is certain to be found in the discharges before the end of abstinence.

More extended discussion of this phenomenon will later be given, for upon it is based a most interesting question in pathology. It suffices here to say that, when the intestinal walls are about freed of old feces, and are in the relaxed condition that results from the processes in operation during the fast, bowel excretion takes the form of an exudation of pathogen from the blood, and this waste is deposited in the form of mucus upon the walls of the intestines. The mucus membrane of the latter in its relaxed state will usually freely slough this coating, especially if peristalsis is stimulated by manipulation of the abdomen and the enema is properly employed. The deposit is discharged, often in formed bodies. An instance recurs in which there came away a mass tubular in shape, eight feet in length, a replica of a portion of the intestinal tract. And often shorter formed sections are discovered. This mucus is viscous, glue-like, in consistency, and, when it disappears, systemic cleansing is near its end.

The more usual indication of disease as it affects body temperature is fever, but in cases of differing temperament, quite frequently after the beginning of a fast, temperature drops a degree or so below normal. This is the result of the absence of food stimulation, for there is nothing inherent in the fast itself that occasions this phenomenon. Even when food is being ingested in cases of long-standing debility temperature is often below register, and in other instances it rises above normal in proportion to the severity of disease. Abstinence from food tends to restore both temperature and pulse to normal, be they high or low at its inception. While the average register of body heat is given at about 98-2/5 degrees Fahrenheit, and the average pulse at about 72 beats to the minute, these figures are not to be regarded as the normal for every organism. There are variations both above and below the standards given that cannot in every instance be considered as arising from disease. A fasting case is here cited in whom, when abstinence was initiated, temperature was constantly at ninety-four degrees; no change was noted until the twentieth day, when an increase of nearly a degree occurred; and average individual normal of ninety-seven degrees was reached ten days later and was thereafter maintained. Here undoubtedly disease was the cause of the abnormally low register observed before the fast, but the norm of the patient in health was subsequently perceived to be slightly below the standard commonly accepted. In a few subjects temperature at the beginning of a fast was so low as not to admit of register upon a clinical thermometer, but invariably normal individual average was reached before the end of treatment Adjustment to standard is likewise attained when fever is a symptom in evidence, and here the change is more rapidly accomplished than when temperature is sub-normal. Body heat, as is seen, has its established tabular measure, and, when it habitually fails by several degrees to reach the common average, the conclusion must be that vitality is deficient. And accompanying sub-normal temperature is always the slow and sluggish pulse, while fever with its raised degrees of heat carries a super-normal heart beat. Of the two pathological states, prognosis in the former is the more favorable. When a condition of extremely low temperature is encountered, hot applications over the spinal column and hot therapeutic baths frequently administered greatly assist in restoring and conserving body heat.

Abnormal temperature and abnormal pulse as well are but symptoms of a pathological condition, and, whether they be high or low, they denote that there is in progress a struggle for life that has little need to be suppressed. If pulse and temperature, either or both, are above or below normal at the beginning of a fast, they will descend or ascend to natural register when disease disappears, or perhaps while some of its symptoms are still displayed. Due to the removal of food stimulation, as has been said, in many instances both temperature and pulse may drop to register slightly below the average shortly after entering upon a fast. And the author lists a few cases with pulse at the beginning of abstinence at about fifty beats to the minute, while one is recorded with the very low rate of twenty-eight. Temperature in these subjects was not, however, sufficiently sub-normal to occasion surprise. While the rates noted in these cases were chronic and most exceptional, they gradually rose to standard for the individuals as the fast progressed to completion.

When the fast is concluded and the body is in the process of rebuilding, a properly balanced vegetarian dietary assures a temperature and pulse with no apparent tendency to rise or fall above individual normal. If, however, the dietetic change has been one from a regimen that formerly included flesh foods to one that is wholly vegetarian in character, pulse register will very probably show a reduction of several counts from its former average.

Several references have heretofore been made to the known absence of hunger in disease. This truth should be self-evident. But additional confirmation is offered in connection with changes of body heat as observed in health and in illness. Physiology asserts and scientific investigation proves that there can be no digestion in the absence of digestive juices, and that there is virtually no secretion of these fluids when body temperature is above normal. Why, then, feed during fever? Without digestion, there can be no nutrition, no upbuilding of tissue structure. Why add the burden of eliminating matter that is not digested, that is useless and noxious excess, to the already extreme effort that nature is making in order to reduce overstimulated heart action and super-normal body heats To correct this condition the only effective measures are to withhold food, to remove the fermenting waste that is causing disease, and to rest those organs that have been functionally unable to cope with tasks beyond their ability to perform. A fever is really a blessing in disguise; it indicates organic activity, which means vitality in reserve. It should never be suppressed, since it is the result of a struggle between the forces of health and disease in which the vital organs will prove the victors if they are correctly, and this means naturally, assisted. Habitually low temperature, on the other hand, predicates organic inactivity, small reserve vitality, a condition that is usually chronic in character, and yet one that admits of improvement under treatment with perhaps surer prospect of correction than do febrile crises in their more extreme forms. But because sub-normal temperature and lowered pulse rate are ordinarily confined to chronic illness, duration of treatment is correspondingly more extended than in those in whom fever and heightened pulse denote acute disease.

Depending upon the physiological tendencies of the individual, after the beginning of a fast and during its several stages, many symptoms not specifically described may develop alone or in combination with others. While some of the phenomena that occur at this time may be ascribed to the depression that succeeds food stimulation, by far the larger number are due to the extreme elimination of body waste in progress. Bowels, kidneys, lungs, and skin are utilized to the limit of their abilities, and, when any one of these means of discharge becomes obstructed because of excess, or has its function impeded because of defect in structure, nature at once seeks another organ to serve as a channel of egress, selecting the latter with no apparent consideration of either its fitness for the service demanded or its ability to perform it. But always the least resistive passage becomes what in this instance may be called the victim.

A few of the simpler symptoms encountered in the earlier stages of fasting have been mentioned, but others more or less common appear in consequence of the unvarying tendency of nature to utilize toxemic elimination paths of least resistance. In some subjects a rash upon the skin occurs; in others a cold with excessive discharge from the nose, bronchial tubes, throat, and eyes is the form in which the results of the purifying process in action is displayed. The salivary glands may excrete in quantity, causing constant expectoration of spittle that may be either fluid or viscous in consistence. The last named functional sign is apt to prove most annoying and disagreeable, so much so that, because of it, fasts at times have been altered in procedure from protracted to interrupted, in order that partial resumption of digestion might change, which in this juncture it never fails to do, the unusual course through which elimination is occurring.

When headaches occur with other symptoms, they are of course due to sudden release of toxic matter, are commonly located in the frontal portion of the brain, and are coincident with the prior stages of abstinence, when the system is accommodating itself to the physiological change of habit then in progress. As purification proceeds, headaches vanish, and in purely functional disturbances the brain experiences more rapid relief than do the organs of the trunk. Connected with headache, in severe functional derangement and when there is organic deficiency, are visual spectra, flashes of white or colored light. And in the graver forms of organic disease a muscular tremor, accompanied with a rotary motion of the eyeball, or even with crossed eyes and faulty vision, sometimes takes place. The latter peculiar variation in symptom has been observed shortly before death, and in extreme form it would seem to indicate approaching dissolution.

Again, partial deafness with humming in the ears is apt to befall. This may ordinarily be relieved locally by careful and constant springing of the inner ears with hot water, assisted by proper manipulation with the tips of the index fingers. This procedure will usually disclose collections of wax, after the removal of which the symptoms disappear. The presence of this secretion at this time in quantity above normal again discloses the extreme of elimination to which the organism is subjected while the function of digestion is suspended. Subjects which, before fasting, have suffered from partial deafness, find this defect much aggravated until the removal of the wax is accomplished and congestion is relieved.

Types that suffer from extreme congestion of the liver or from obstruction of the upper portion of the small intestines may intermittently experience contraction of the muscles of the hands and arms with cramping pains—the legs are rarely affected. Local relief may here be obtained through hand vibration and deep manipulation along the spinal column in its cervical and upper dorsal regions.

Emaciation in the fast cannot properly be regarded as a symptom pathologic in origin. It is the result of the elimination of toxic substances from the system, and there is also a loss occasioned by the use by cell organism, and by brain and nerves, of the reserve-pabulum stored in the interstices of tissue. Diminution in weight due to the latter reason is, however, slight in comparison with that arising from toxemic elimination. It may be stated that wasting of the body is usually greater in cases in whom organic atrophy or cirrhosis exists than in those who suffer otherwise from disease, but, in a fast, loss of weight is proportionately less in the instances referred to than it is in the presence of functional disease or of organic hypertrophy.

In his *True Science of Living* Dr. Edward Hooker Dewey quotes from Yeo's *Physiology* a table purporting to show the estimated loss of the several tissues of the body in instances of starvation. The table follows:

Fat	91%
Muscle	30%
Liver	56%
Spleen	63%
Blood	17%
Brain and Nerve Centers	0%

Dr. Dewey terms this table, "Nature's Bill of Fare for the Sick," assuming that, in the absence of ingested food, both in fasting and in starving, the body is supported upon the tissues lost. It is natural and correct to infer that a portion of this missing material is in the circumstances utilized in the maintenance of cell structure, but by far the larger portion of it is purely waste, is matter that is not constructive but pathogenic. As is shown in the chapter dealing with death during fasting, there is no certainty that the proportions given in the table above result in all instances. One point, however, is observed as constant and invariable—the brain and the nerve centers with their branches are never reduced in structure nor in quality, notwithstanding the duration of the period of abstinence, unless in themselves they are organically diseased.

Delirium in disease is not always to be regarded as an alarming symptom. Temporary conditions of mental aberration apparent in confusion of thought, incoherency of speech, and, in some instances, unconsciousness, are characteristic of certain constitutions whenever body temperature rises above a fixed point. This, possibly, is an inherited tendency, for, on the other hand, there are many temperaments who retain control of the mind in any and all forms of disease, when the brain itself is not the seat of disturbance. In the treatment of disease that is functional in origin, it is rarely the case that delirium occurs during a fast, but, it may, and, if it does, its appearance is due to extreme auto-intoxication from waste deposited in the intestinal tract and not evacuated with sufficient rapidity. If delirium be present at all, it will occur when the process of elimination is at its height, and it will cease as suddenly as it began, when the cause of the toxemia has been removed from the bowels. If proper preparation for the fast has been observed, this symptom will never appear in cases of purely functional derangement. But it may appear if a fast is broken before purification of the system has been attained, or, if the patient is given food in amount beyond the capability of his organs to digest, when feeding is resumed at the end of a completed fast. In cases when abstinence from food is forced and involuntary, as for example in shipwreck and mine accident, delirium, if it occur, results from the mental strain attendant upon the situation, and it, together with the mortality that may happen, could often be obviated were knowledge of the resources of the human body more general. In organic disease, before a fast or while it endures, delirium may last for some time, and, while its first cause is one with that in functional trouble, its persistence is due to defects in organism that prevent elimination. And, even though recovery be possible, these cases are most obstinate in yielding to treatment, since the process of purification is exceedingly slow in accomplishment, while recuperation is similarly delayed. This type of patient requires more care and caution in handling than does any other, for the sufferer, losing faith in the power of nature to overcome the condition, is apt to lose courage as well. Resort to food and to drugs may be made, and the outcome, doubtful before, is now almost inevitably fatal. When one is confronted by this situation, the lesson to be learned is that of recognition of organic limitation, for while the very functioning of an organ diseased has a tendency to restore that organ to normal action, it must be remembered and emphasized that special function in the physical body is capable only of operating within bounds, beyond which lies disaster.

A fast properly conducted can never cause delirium nor affect the mental processes other than favorably. Much of insanity is the result of congestion-producing functional disorder, and this sort of mental aberration is ordinarily followed by complete restoration to normal reasoning power after a fast more or less protracted in length has been scientifically administered.

A general classification of the symptom of disease that tends towards limiting the appearance of certain signs to certain ailments can never be made with accuracy. It is true that the science of medicine labels and catalogues all symptoms, and that it is its plan to await development before announcing diagnosis. But the science of medicine, neglecting or ignoring cause, seemingly devotes its entire attention to the suppression of manifestation, and classification of symptoms upon the basis adopted finds items overlapping in such manner as to make distinction difficult if not impossible. An arrangement of disease forms may, however, be made in a general way along lines that are more or less sharply defined.

1.—Ailments purely functional in origin that readily yield to natural treatment. In these cases, because of accumulation of waste in the digestive tract and in tissue, organs are hampered in function but are in nowise structurally disabled nor in themselves diseased.

Here gradual improvement is noted from the beginning of preparation for a fast, and recovery is always to be anticipated.

2.—Organic defect in slight degree, occasioning disturbance because of work inefficiently performed by an organ that is partially disabled. This condition places heavier burdens upon other organs and functionally unbalances the entire system. During the progess of a fast disagreeable symptoms are noted in these cases, and it is possible that full functional power may never be restored. However, if structural defect has not reached the degree that denotes inclusion in the class following, and, if care be exercised during the time of convalescence, recovery is usually assured.

3.—Organic defect of such degree that the functioning of a vital organ is rendered impossible or nearly so. A gradual decline, beginning before the fast and continuing with a short interval of relief after entering upon abstinence, is the characteristic indication. Relief noted may be such as to inspire hope of recovery, but, if the condition be as stated, there is no possibility of cure.

In cases of disease purely functional in character, the fasting patient usually discovers after the first general symptoms disappear, that his strength has apparently increased, and that he is able to attend to ordinary duty without difficulty and with marvelously clear mentality. In other words, with the loss of stimulation due to food poison, disease subsides, and real strength becomes manifest. The patient is not less weak nor more strong than at any time during his previous diseased state when living under toxic stimulation. but the fast has served to uncover his true condition and to demonstrate that a sick man is not of necessity a weak man. It should now be quite clear to the reader that in disease many or the avenues through which energy is normally released are so obstructed by cumulative waste and its effects as partially to prevent the expression of vital force, and that, in the early stages of illness, weakness is but inability to assert latent strength.

The subject of food stimulation has not received the attention that it deserves in any system of therapeutics, for it is always an important factor to be considered both in health and in disease. When the body has become accustomed to a dietetic regimen, fixed in quantity and in hours of ingestion, it strenuously rebels when denied. The system may be greatly overfed; it may slowly be poisoning itself through its own indiscretions; yet the omission of a meal puts appetite into action. Given the usual quota, metabolism of a sort continues until excess proves too heavy a burden to be carried, or some micro-organism finds environment suitable for multiplication and growth; then nature calls a halt and attempts correction through her only remedy, disease. Recuperation begins when the accustomed stimulus, food, is withdrawn, but the subject is plunged into the depths. Stimulation, so long a habit, now seems necessary to counteract the depression caused by deprivation, and to the latter is added fear, engendered by tradition, that nourishment is needful to foster strength, and even that death through starvation will shortly occur. Here mentality must be called to the rescue, and the will must be asserted in order to avert apprehension and with it the desire to resume the ingestion of food.

Careful study of the symptoms of disease, as they occur when either feeding or fasting is the rule, reveals the law through which nature works to restore a diseased body to health. It may briefly be given as a process of systemic elimination, upon lines of least resistance, of toxin-producing substances retained in the intestinal canal or in tissue. The signs of distress, the symptoms, may often be locally relieved by the application of heat, water, sunlight, air, manipulation, or other natural means, but disease can never be eradicated through mere suppression of symptom. It must be dealt with at its source; and, despite its variety of expression, it has but one cause, digestion, with nutrition, inefficiently performed, and but one remedy, systemic elimination of the toxins resulting therefrom.

In the process of treatment outlined in the text frequent examination of the discharges of the body are made. These in connection with other indications give an index of the progress of systemic purification. Both urine and feces are methodically tested, chemically and microscopically, and the nature of the products of elimination is thus determined. In the prior days of fasting the urine is invariably high in color and in specific gravity, and its reaction is usually strongly acid, while urea, phosphates and other mineral salts, and bilious products are present in abundance. When the first flush of elimination subsides, specific gravity is much lowered (it may register below 1.010), and mineral substances decrease in quantity. If treatment excluded the daily enemas and baths, if it were confined solely to abstinence from food, specific gravity of the urine would at first quickly rise and would continue to be high in register, but, because of prompt removal of waste from the colon by means of the enema, and because of dilution of the fluids of the body through absorption of water through the walls of the bowel, density of urine is diminished, hence its lighter specific gravity. When purification nears completion, reaction of urine may assume a neutral or even an alkaline character, which again will change to slight acid upon resumption of ingestion.

Even in the early years of life systematic overloading of the system with food is responsible for high arterial pressure. And the supertension of later existence is in large measure preventable through dietetic care in youth and middle age in determining systemic condition, tests of blood pressure are valuable, and they should frequently be made during treatment. One of the salutary consequences obtained by means of a fast is that blood pressure, like temperature and pulse, is uniformly brought to normal for the individual. This is an invariable result whether register be lower or higher than average when treatment begins. But the same notation must again be made that was commented upon when temperature and pulse were under discussion: tabulated average register cannot be regarded as fixed for differing organisms, since variations both above and below standard occur that cannot be attributed in every instance to disease. In this, as in other respects, each individual possesses a norm of his own. It may be stated, however, that, when systemic cleansing is accomplished, this norm is usually lower in register than the previous tabulated standard. In the matured body, with but little differences noted as age increases, a general normal in blood pressure ranges about 120 for the systolic, with about 80 as the diastolic register. This of course supposes the subject to be subsisting upon non-stimulative food material.

9

Difficulties Encountered in Fasting

Drugs Cause Organic Troubles:

Scientists Quoted on Fasting:

Auto-Intoxication

One of the most serious obstacles to general acceptance of the fast as a therapeutic measure by both the public and the medical profession is the innate subconscious element of fear engendered by orthodox dicta that nourishment must be supplied lest vitality fail. Man must eat, sick or well, "to keep up strength." The degree to which this conception is fallacious may be gathered from the text; yet very recently medical science has "discovered" the efficacy of "short fasts" in the treatment of diabetes and in the reduction of obesity. Prediction is made that eventually all of the information gathered upon the therapeusis of the fast by those who, like the author, have devoted years of service to the task, will be adopted and claimed as original by the dominant cult.

It is unfortunate that enthusiasm produced by the beneficial effects of personal trial of abstinence from food for food for the relief of disease has caused the recipients of these benefits to rush into print, detailing their experiences and advising other sufferers to go and do likewise. In greater part the articles and books referred to have been written by men incompetent of understanding more than the mere results obtained in their own individual cases; and the consequences of such ill advised essays into unfamiliar fields are obvious. Regardless of the rationale of the method, and ignorant of the physiological changes that the administration of a fast involves, other inexperienced hands undertake the treatment without guidance, with the result that in many instances harm to the patient succeeds, with consequent unmerited adverse criticism of the method.

In the milder instances of functional illness no possible harm can result when food is omitted for one or for several days, provided the needful aids to elimination are employed. But protracted fasting in the absence of skilful, scientific guidance is, as indicated, fraught with the probability of injury to one who has the temerity to undertake the experience acting upon his own impulse.

If human bodies continued to exist from birth in the usually normal organic condition they then possess, the fast applied when functional disturbance occurs in all probability would proceed to its logical end without difficulty. But, through constant wrong living, through chronic abuse of the vital processes, through lowered muscular tone and consequent impedence of nerve force, and through the effects of symptomatic suppression by drug dosage, the average adult acquires defects in organic structure.

In infancy, when functional disease develops, a drug is given for the suppression of the symptom, and virtually always nourishment is supplied. Two errors in treatment are here noted—the administration of a substance reputed to possess properties that will remedy, that is, suppress, the symptom leaving the cause of the disturbance to take care of itself; and the ingestion of food by an organism which, because of disease, is incapable of digesting the same. The results are that in many instances the children die; in others, functional paralysis of portions of the alimentary tract is caused; in still others, the resistive powers of the infant are such as to permit it to survive, despite both dosage and the administration of food. Yet in the latter event harm rather than benefit derives, and, since the evil is done during the growing period, retardation of organic development occurs, and in future years disease symptoms arise at the points affected in infancy.

Careful observation of thousands of fasting subjects gives proof that a scientifically conducted fast will result in the correction of all ailments that are functional in cause, but that it can never, either through the effects of itself or of its auxiliaries, wholly overcome organic defects. However, the fast will do this—it will uncover the condition of the system, and, if defects or deficiencies exist, it will cause their nature to be clearly displayed. It is in effect an infallible diagnostic expedient.

One whose organs are functionally equal to the requirements of elimination undergoes a period of abstinence from food with no severe distressing symptoms. And, when unusual manifestations occur, it is virtually certain that in some degree defects in organism lie within the body. Post mortem examination of subjects who died while a fast was in progress has given convincing evidence upon this point, and it has further demonstrated that in these cases death would have happened whether the patient were fasting or feeding. To this may be added the observation that, because of lessened organic labor, life in the instances referred to was for a time prolonged. But there are cases in whom distressing symptoms appear as results of organic deficiency which has not yet progressed to an incurable state. These cases may, under proper guidance, hope for relief that may prove permanent.

A drug with regard to its effects upon the animal body may be said to be any substance that will influence metabolism—the continuous process by which living cells undergo chemical change. Hence a drug also influences the functioning of the vital organs. According to this definition foods, even though they be excellent in quality and reasonable in quantity, react as drugs upon the organism. That is to say, food both influences metabolism and the functioning of the vital organs. But food is not necessarily poisonous in its effects as are all substances ordinarily classified as drugs; yet it is easily seen that, if taken in too great quantity, if not properly combined, if ingested when hunger is absent or when emotion is aroused, or if it be unwholesome in quality, food will act as poison upon tissue and upon organic function. In like manner substances formed within the body from the process of tissue waste may act as do drugs upon living cells. This occurs when elimination is inadequate, and hence arise the auto-toxins, through the effects of which systemic resistance, that is, immunity from disease, is reduced, and the way opened for the large group of so-called infectious maladies.

It cannot be fairly assumed that, upon dissecting a body after death, lesions that are present in any organ are due solely to previous drugging. Where two such agencies as disease and drugs have been simultaneously acting upon a living organism, it is difficult, in the absence of a standard, to decide whether a specific result is due to one, or to the other, or to both. But it is a significant fact that, in every instance of death occurring during a fast as recorded in the writer's experience, each of the subjects, with but a single exception, had been drugged in early life, and that the effects of this dosage upon vital organs and tissue, as shown in arrested development and in structural change, were precisely such as could and would have been caused by an active poison. Preponderance of evidence gathered from the findings of these autopsies makes for the presence at some period previous to death of some toxic substance, some active noxious agent, that permanently and harmfully affected tissue structure.

The constant use of drugs to suppress the symptoms of disease in the growing child not only lowers physical resistance but it also retards the development of the vital organs, which in some instances suffer permanent deformation. Yet, despite this handicap, the framework of the body eventually reaches normal adult dimension. The disparity presented by organs in whole or in part nearly infantile in size functioning in a body adult in proportion necessarily causes forms of distress that will assuredly end in chronic disease, since the undersized organs are not equal to the demands made upon them. The process that is predominant when a fast is in progress is that of elimination, and it is easy to understand that, in a body in which, for instance, portions of the intestinal tract are under dimension, or in which one or other of the organs of special function is structurally imperfect, the labor of ridding the system of accumulated waste is beyond the ability of the organism perfectly to accomplish. Therefore, to the degree in which organic defects exist is determined the severity of the struggle with disease. In other words, the effort which is being made to east out from the body gathered impurity becomes proportionately more difficult when organic imperfections are present. In the normally developed adult body chronic disease or drugs may produce like effects, but here vital organs are of full dimension, and results are shown, not in arrested development, but wholly in structural tissue-change.

Whenever, because of organs functionally incapacitated for any reason, the products of food and tissue waste cannot be evacuated through proper channels, general poisoning of the blood stream occurs. The resulting condition is known as auto-intoxication, or toxemia, referred to previously as a state of unbalance when both secretion and excretion are checked and the blood is surcharged with waste to the degree of developing a crisis or acute disease. This state gives rise in the subject to manifestations that may become alarming. The brain may be affected to the extent of mild delirium, hiccoughs persistent in character may occur, or the patient may sink into stupor; and there are other forms which the symptoms may take that will cause distress. In a fast that has been correctly approached toxemia so intense in degree can never arise. But if, as happens when inexperienced direction is given, food is discontinued abruptly, accessories are omitted, and no preparatory period of dieting is observed, symptoms as mentioned are apt to be manifested. Even when all essentials are correctly followed, slight toxemia may be present in cases that are fasting, when these are sufferers from chronic functional disease or from some structural organic defect. But, if the subject has been prepared for the period of abstinence in the manner heretofore described, and, if the hygienic accessories of treatment are consistently employed, symptoms that are distressing are not likely to occur.

The presence of toxins in the body is for the most part attributable to inability of the eliminative organs to perform their work. For some cause or other the latter do not dispose of waste in amount sufficient to balance intake or production. When difficulty is encountered in disposing of the refuse produced progressively during a fast, lack of eliminative power is its causation, and this arises from nerve force impeded through impingement of vertebrae, from structural organic defect, from lesions caused by previous drugging, or from waste production so extreme that even normal organs are unable to cope with it.

The physician who holds the concept that disease and cure are a unity is not at all concerned with the presence or absence of the various toxins, nor by the symptoms in evidence, save as they act as indices of the functioning ability of vital organs. If the latter are in normal structural condition, the products of food in excess of need may interfere with function because of simple congestion, which we have seen is easily relieved. But the vital parts of the human body are in many instances structurally defective through drug dosage or through food stimulation, and these organs may in consequence be brought into action only by the administration of additional drugs or by further stimulus. In these circumstances elimination can take place only abnormally, with in all cases but partial removal of body waste. In treating disease by natural methods the character of the toxin is not considered excepting in so far as it is an indication of the severity of illness, and the thought paramount concerns the condition of the organs involved, with their ability to function, rather than with the nature of the circulating poison.

The toxication or poisoning that results from absorption of certain products of metabolism has been said sometimes to cause delirium in the subject. This phenomenon, because it has infrequently been observed while a fast was in progress, has given rise to the contention that protracted abstinence from food occasions insanity. Nothing can be further from truth, for, when toxic elimination has been successfully accomplished, when the system is fully and physiologically purified, mentality is at maximum; and, on the other hand, cases displaying mental aberration to toxemia caused by overfeeding are speedily brought to sanity when food is denied. In fact, extreme auto-intoxication occurs more frequently when the subject is feeding than when he is fasting, and an overfed system is productive of poisons the effects of which upon mentality are more serious and more lasting than are those of stimulants or narcotics.

Wounds and broken bones are healed and united by natural processes, and it is only through the operation of the latter that cures may be achieved. The fast and its accessories are not in themselves "processes", as the term is here used. Their office is that of the removal of obstacles that lie in the paths of action invariably pursued by nature in effecting her purpose of systemic cleansing, of casting out of the body the poisons that are the source of its disease. As a result of restoration of function that follows a successful fast instances do occur where organic structural break-down is arrested and the organ is again placed in functioning condition, but these instances are exceptional. However, undertaking a fast in the hope that it in itself will succeed in overcoming to the point of recovery serious structural organic defects, wounds, and broken bones, is to hope for an absurdity. In these circumstances the benefits that accrue from the application of the method are proportioned to the degree of the power of the organ or of the tissue involved to recover itself.

Death during a fast cannot occur unless there is organic disease, and not then unless the organ or organs affected are in such degenerated state as not to permit of repair; and it is conclusively demonstrated that in a scientifically directed fast, although death in the conditions cited cannot be averted, yet because of organic labor lessened, life is prolonged for days or weeks, and distress and pain, if present, are much alleviated.

The differentiation between starvation and fasting is made herein upon the basis that starvation occurs in consequence of food being denied to a system that is in need of sustenance, and that fasting consists in intentional abstinence from food by a system in disease, a system which in consequence of its physical unbalance is not only without desire for nutriment, but which in reality is in no need of it until its organism is purified and again in condition to perform its functions normally. The distinction stated may be admitted, yet the fact is not altered that the two processes are in essence largely identical. But it has been observed that, deposited within the body, lies a reserve store of aliment, and it is also to be observed that this reserve is not in the main utilized for tissue rebuilding, but is in most part intended at all times for the support and maintenance of the nervous system; and it is only when this supply of nerve sustenance is exhausted or prevented from serving its purpose that starvation occurs. Because of the possibility of these happenings in disease, the body may starve though it is well fed, for often in instances of overfeeding there is mal-assimilation, often an essential organ is rendered functionally incapable through congestion, in consequence of which the nervous system is hindered from consuming its necessary nourishment since the channels of supply are obstructed. Hence it should be apparent that in functional disease during a fast starvation can begin only when fasting ends—at the disappearance of disease, at the return of hunger.

Whether we regard the vital principle, the animating force of the animal body, as an entity or, as modern science would have it, as the result of chemical transformations, it must be agreed that, during a fast whatever tissue construction occurs happens in consequence of nutriment supplied from the reserve noted above, and this Dr. E. H. Dewey termed "Nature's bill of fare for the sick." Deprived of food, the subject then must subsist upon this menu, details of which have already been given in the table quoted from Yeo's *Physiology*, a table which shows the estimated losses of the several tissues of the body in cases of starvation. During periods of abstinence from food the organism then subsists upon itself, and loss of body weight must occur. Directly this loss is due to the elimination, first, of the waste that caused disease, and, next and continuously with the other, of the refuse produced by catabolism or cell destruction. The dominant process in action at this time is that of expulsion of disease-producing matter, and it is obvious that the latter is at no point available for the repair of tissue, and that, held within the system, it acts not only obstructively in the avenues of vitality, but that it also toxically vitiates function. This is true of all refuse retained in the organism at any time, for this material, because of delay in expulsion, is rendered harmful through putrefactive changes.

The points of difficulty related heretofore are in a sense technical in character, but there are objections which embody personal opinion and prejudice that at times develop into serious obstacles. While fasting for the relief of disease has been known and practiced individually in all countries of the world from prehistoric times, it was never advanced in any land to the point where it could be regarded as a distinct system of therapeutics until the decade beginning about fifty years ago. Its rise from sporadic application to the dignity of a school occurred about that time in the United States, and from then on its exponents and practitioners, persisting in the face of scientific opposition, gradually accomplished their purpose by proving their contentions, and at length have the satisfaction of seeing their conclusions accepted and adopted without apology or acknowledgment by what may be termed intellectual authority.

There is no form of ignorance that is so difficult to

overcome and to instruct as is of the "scientific" mind. And, when the latter, as it sometimes does, obtains a conception of its error, it is extremely loath to admit, first, that it has not always been in possession of the truth, and, second, that it should render due credit to the mind responsible for its change of concept or belief. And, if the position of the individual be such that he may with authority employ the power of mere assertion, it is usually much the easier way to announce as one's own discovery that which formerly one has denied and condemned, perhaps through prejudice, but more often through sheer ignorance.

In this connection quotations are made from several articles and books recently issued by medical authors. These screeds are given with small comment, but they serve to illustrate the contemptuous attitude assumed by those of whom Louis Kuhne years ago said this: "Everywhere the new science of healing finds sympathetic acceptance, except among a few skeptics and those who believe that they know everything better than anyone else, and who generally consider it superfluous to make practical trial of any method strange to the tenets of their own."

First let us hear Dr. W. A. Evans, who writes *How to Keep Well,* a syndicated letter at present published daily in various newspapers throughout the country. Dr. Evans has this to say about fasting:

"On the shelves of the Crerar Library (Chicago), or any other library of similar equipment, are many books on fasting. I know none that is even half way scientific, nor a quarter way trustworthy. One reason for this is that fasting is the sport of amateurs, as one writer calls it. He might have added that it is the fad of faddists and the field of the faker. To further complicate matters, it is all mixed up with religion. Every religion has always had religious feasts, which are gorges, and its fasts.

"Prof. Morgulis of the University of Nebraska has just put out a truly scientific book on the subject. The only trouble about this book is that it is so accurate, scientific, and technical that the man who needs it most cannot understand it.

"Fasting is a remedial agent of enormous power—power for good and power for harm. Nothing the doctor carries in his saddle bags approximates fasting in its therapeutic possibilities. In fact, a doctor attends a patient through a long illness, giving him four kinds of medicine four times every day, it is probable that the under-nutrition through which the patient has passed by reason of his loss of appetite, vomiting, diarrhea, or other quality of his disease, or the dieting to which he was subjected, influenced both the patient and his disease far more than did the medicine which was given.

Comes now Dr. Frederick M. Allen, A. B., M. D., of the Rockefeller Institute Hospital, who about the year, 1915, advanced his "discovery" of the "starvation treatment" of diabetes. There is no need to devote more time to him than to say that as far back as 1878

Dr. Edward Hooker Dewey successfully employed the fast in treating diabetes mellitus.

A quotation now follows from *Fasting and Undernutrition*, the book of Professor Morgulis of the University of Nebraska College of Medicine. This is the author mentioned by Dr. Evans, who attributes to the Professor the only scientific work written upon the fast—so scientific in fact that the man who needs it most cannot understand it. In his book Professor Morgulis has devoted himself solely to the physiological aspect of abstinence from food with its effects upon animals in health, neglecting its therapeutical possibilities, excepting to say in his preface:—"In the hands of the skilful *practitioner of medicine* total abstinence from food may prove a wonderfully effective weapon in restoring health. The therapeutic value of inanition, however, should be studied experimentally and not be left to the judgment of amateur enthusiasts. The practical value of inanition will never be fully utilized until both laymen and the medical profession lose their instinctive fear of fasting". (My italics.) Professor Morgulis, scientific in mind and expression though he may be, makes in the statement given the egregious error of confusing inanition, starvation, with fasting, forgetting or perhaps not knowing that there is no malnutrition comparable to the starvation that accompanies overeating.

Quotations from the writings of these men of science are made thus at length for several reasons. It is desired that the reader may be impressed with the truth that fasting for therapeutic purposes—fasting for the prevention and relief of disease—has been known and practiced for all of the historic ages of man. It is also to be emphasized that all animate nature, save man, instinctively refuses food when physical balance is disturbed. And, whether the discussion conducted herein be from the standpoint of science "scientific" or not, it will stand the sole test that makes for truth in that the results connoted are based upon long, faithful, and accurate observation and experiment of minds as capable of receiving and recording the phenomena connected with abstinence from food in illness or in health as are those of the scientists quoted. And it should possess the further distinction of being easily understandable by him who needs it most.

The premises of the argument underlying the application of a fast for therapeutic will bear repetition. Disease, in whatever form evidenced, whatever the symptom displayed, has its origin at the threshold of digestion. In disease itself lies relief. Disease and cure, viewed from the standpoint of nature, are a unity. The former may not be suppressed lest the latter fail of attainment. When an organism, constituted as is the body of man, becomes the victim of its own violation of hygienic law, when the avenues through which vital force, the source of life, is transmitted, are permitted to become obstructed, unless these channels are cleansed, are opened for the passage of energy, life ceases and death occurs. In order that the passages through which the life principle reaches the separate parts of the human body may be free and unobstructed, a system of elimination exists. Building of tissue—assimilation—takes place as the result of food ingested and digested, but health depends upon a balance between nutrition and elimination. And there is no eliminative agency known to science comparable with a properly administered fast.

Dr. Evans has said that the book of Professor Morgulis is a treatise upon the fast that is truly scientific. And there is no doubt that *Fasting and, Undernutrition* is a thesis most carefully prepared and couched in purely scientific terms. But it deals entirely with inanition in healthy animals and with a few short fasts undertaken by healthy human professionals. Fasting in health and fasting when disease is in evidence are two distinct processes, and the writer believes that even science must concede differing chemical transformations and reactions in sickness and in health. And further, because the results of many years of observation, experiment, and induction are placed before students in terms that are easily understandable, it must not be concluded that the truths discovered and related are non-scientific and are to be discarded as fallacies. Yet the professed scientist is most free in offering the sort of criticism mentioned and inferred, and this has its weight with those who are subservient to intellectual authority, with those who are either unwilling or incapable of thinking for themselves.

It is thus seen that obstacles are put in the way of the practice of fasting as a therapeutic measure by the scientist and by the ignorant layman, but this has a direct advantage in promoting investigation, for criticism, especially from scientific sources, necessarily induces in an intelligent and conscientious observer intense concentration upon all phases of the subject. No point that may conduce to favorable issue is overlooked; no natural law or accessory is permitted to remain without investigation. Considerations merely selfish in character might here prove motives for a certain sort of endeavor—desire for gain, the hope of triumphing over other schools. But a broader deeper feeling actuates the true student of nature In him the search for perfect understanding of cause and effect, the giving of a truth to the world the relief of physical suffering, are the stimuli that impel him to surmount the obstacles he meets and that bring success to his labors.

The discovery of the general therapeutic worth of the fast was soon followed by a knowledge of its value as a diagnostic agent. Properly directed, the method never fails to uncover every weak point in an ailing body, to reveal the exact location of organic distress or defect, the focal point of disease. Continued experiment and observation established the desirability of correct approach to complete abstinence from food through gradual diminution of intake, thus insuring systemic accommodation to the physiological changes involved, while permitting elimination naturally to dominate. Here also was demonstrated the importance of enemata and cleansing baths for the purpose of facilitating the disposal of the harmful products of catabolism.

During a fast, as elimination of body waste progresses,

the observer is permitted, to a degree approaching accuracy, to determine the condition of function of each vital organ, and, if structural defect is present, it is certain to be detected. For cessation of food intake inhibits organic labor with the exception of that compelled by systemic utilization of the reserve contained in tissue. At this time organs, the functioning ability of which is equal to normal demand, completely relax with no symptoms of distress and with no signs of defect in structure; while organs diseased, either functionally or structurally, maintain a state of congestion combined with distress or pain, the latter due to inflammatory conditions or to lesions already formed. In addition, the internal chemistry of the organism is more or less fully and accurately revealed, since discharges from the body are most easily analyzed, unmixed as they are with the products of recently ingested food.

In the event that grave organic defect exists in a patient, signs more or less determinant are displayed both during the time of preparation and in the early stages of a fast. Serious symptoms do not as a rule transpire until about the second or third week of abstinence, and then these demonstrations may assume any of the forms of debility. In the experience of the writer are several cases in whom at this period violent delirium occurred, as well as others who suffered from milder mental derangement. But in all of these instances, even in those in which death succeeded, there was rapid emergence from the mental cloud, and consciousness continued unimpaired either to dissolution or to recovery.

In the cases mentioned as having developed extreme mental disturbance some structural deformation of the colon was noted. This defect, despite the employment of high enemata, acted as an obstacle to the movement of bowel contents through the organ, and the refuse, liquid in form, purely waste and poisonous in the extreme, was thus permitted to be absorbed in quantity, giving rise to a degree of toxemia that induced the delirium. No surprise is evinced at intoxication resulting from the consumption of alcohol; none should be shown at the drunkenness produced by poisons that are self-generated.

There are other instances in whom organic development of the small intestines has been arrested in early life through disease or through drugs, or in whom other forms of deformation of this portion of the alimentary tract exist. During a fast these subjects may exhibit distressing symptoms that continue for some days. They seldom, however, experience mental crises, but they do require exceeding care in direction, both while fasting and in the after-period of rebuilding. But always each case develops its own manifestations, and it does not necessarily follow that severe forms of mental aberration invariably proceed from intestinal organic defect.

When functional disease alone is the difficulty to be overcome, the case in treatment is simplicity itself. Patients of this class ordinarily are able to care for themselves throughout a fast of the duration necessary. But, whenever organic disease exists, whether in the form presented in Class 2, or in that in Class 3 of previous mention (Chapter VIII), unpleasant and possibly severe symptoms are inevitable. In these circumstances all of the courage and the wisdom evolved through long experience in handling disease as nature dictates are needed to meet the conditions. Knowledge of the direct causation of the delirium, of the stupor, of any and all of the symptoms of toxic poisoning, none of which are ever wholly absent in extreme organic disability, then gives confidence to the directing mind. *It knows that, because of abstinence from food, because of the purifying processes in progress, because of reduced organic effort, the life of the patient will be considerably prolonged. It also knows that, if death occur, it is the result of lesions in the organ or organs involved, progressed to a degree that even the minimized labor demanded is beyond performance.*

Let it be repeated that in the fast there can be no danger of death by starvation. The safeguard of all life is hunger—true hunger, not appetite. And, when the process of systemic purification is successfully completed—and this is always possible unless conditions just noted are existent—hunger must return and food must be supplied.

Skill in the treatment of disease by the use of the fast and its natural accessories cannot be acquired from books, for as yet there are none that cover any except basic truths, and these with but meager detail. The subject is vast, and it is the more interesting in that it controverts age-long belief in the efficacy of drugs and the efficiency of the medicine men, the opposition of whom to the spread of its teaching is still most effective. Hence only long practice of the method with resulting experience can give the knowledge essential in surmounting the difficulties that may and do arise.

In concluding this chapter it is again affirmed that the fast in itself is but a means to an end' a process that permits of organic rest, physiological purification, and bodily recuperation. Cure—recovery—cannot be achieved until the subject agrees then and thereafter to cooperate with nature thus permitting her to carry what has been successfully begun to successful conclusion.

The Duratin of the Fast 10

Distinction between Appetite and Hunger:

The Law of Hunger Determines the Length of a Fast

The Duration of a fast to complete purification is a matter that can never be predicated in any individual case, for the beginning of the period of abstinence from food is coincidental with illness, and the end is reached, in the absence of organic deficiency, when hunger marks the return of digestive power. Until true hunger becomes apparent, and it cannot be mistaken, a fast which has for its purpose full systemic cleansing should continue. Not until hunger indicates the need for food is the organism in condition to receive and transform it into tissue structure.

The sensation of hunger is a safeguard established by nature to insure bodily maintenance. It is the first faculty that the infant exercises after birth, and its office in all life is that of a watchful caretaker entrusted with interests beyond the ordinary in import. Natural consciousness of hunger has largely been usurped by appetite, by artificial craving produced by the cultivation of the sense of taste and by regularity in the habits of feeding. Hunger is an involuntary sensation —as involuntary as is the beating of the heart. It is not created by the individual, nor does it make its appearance at stated hours or by exercise of the will. Hunger, the law that governs the conservation of all physical life, is constructive; but appetite, its counterfeit, easily called into being, and just as easily caused to appear at fixed times, is destructive in effect.

In disease hunger is absent; and during fasting appetite, too, ordinarily vanishes after a few days. When, in the fast, toxic elimination is complete, hunger, not appetite, returns. Hunger is normal; appetite is abnormal. And this distinction, considered in connection with the breaking of a fast, is most important. The question of resumption of feeding does not lie for answer in the judgment of either physician or patient. It rests with the law of hunger alone. During a fast that is to be prolonged until hunger returns, food of any kind is an intruder, for the energy of the body is being directed through the organs of elimination towards cleansing the system of self-manufactured poison. The coated tongue, the foul breath, all of the more or less unpleasant symptoms heretofore described, are but signs of the presence in decomposing condition of food and tissue waste. And, being of decomposition, they are also signs of the death of life-giving substances and of portions of the organism itself, the products of which are most harmful unless promptly removed from the body. When toxic elimination has reached the vanishing point, the juncture at which rebuilding of cell structure is demanded lest the body die, hunger will definitively appear. Hunger is the abiding law of animal existence; it is the signal of instinct by which the living organism perceives that food is needed for repair and growth. And, in a fast, with it, the clean tongue, the sweet breath, the signs of normal life, are coincident.

In functional disease a fast may be carried to its logical end without anxiety, for resident in the body there exists at all times a supply of tissue pabulum for use in repair and growth, whether the latter be ordinary or extraordinary. This reserve is constantly called upon in health or in illness, while feeding or fasting, for the nourishment and upbuilding of nerve and brain substances, and the latter never suffer deterioration in quality nor in structure unless in themselves they are specifically diseased. Even in instances of death from starvation, nerve tissue and that of the brain show no loss. They make use of the food reserve held in the interstices of tissue, and they draw upon this accumulation for support. The nervous system regains its energy, when depleted, through rest alone, but it maintains its quality through the means described. Hence, so long as there remain tissues, and this includes the blood, sufficient to carry on the work of the functions

.nd of the circulation, brain and nerves will continue their directing tasks, and they cannot waste in the process.

That a supply of healthy tissue food exists within the body during a fast, and that it is not exhausted until the return of natural hunger, does not rest for proof upon the dictum of medical observation in cases of starvation. In the chapter of the text devoted to illustrative cases an instance is cited of eventual healing by first intention during a fast of fifty-two days of a sore three inches in diameter, a suppurating sore so virulent in character that the periosteum of the bone beneath was exposed. Two cases of illness during pregnancy are also noted in which the prospective mothers fasted for twenty-two and thirty days respectively. In the bodies of each of these women the growth of the fetus was progressive and normal, despite omission of ingestion. Due to their functional disorder, hunger was absent in these pregnant patients, but a supply of nourishment, and wholesome nourishment at that, was at hand, and it served to maintain the organisms of the mothers and to build those of the forming children for the periods given above, and at term each mother was delivered of a child in all respects physiologically normal.

The signs of a successfully completed fast are most easily recognized. The tongue is pink and clean, the breath is sweet, and appetite or false hunger is supplanted by natural desire for food, a sensation that is exquisite beyond description, and that may be realized only by a purified and regenerated system.

Again, because of the importance of the subject, iteration is made. Hunger is at all times to be distinguished from appetite. Hunger is discriminative and preserves the body. Appetite is abnormal desire and ultimately destroys. Hunger is primarily indicated in the mouth, and, if not relieved, it becomes an organic craving that can be satisfied only by digestible food; but appetite cannot be so silenced; it continually searches for this or for that; it is never satisfied.

Natural hunger indicates a system with all channels of vitality freed from obstruction, with every nerve sensitized to the extreme of response to impulse. This adjustment of bodily power and function is invariably evident when a fast has been scientifically conducted to completion. And it is here observed that this conserved of the organism, this all-important warder of its needs, stands ever in the guise of what may be termed organic intelligence, for, in a body free from toxin-producing substances, hunger displays selective intelligence, in great part demanding foods adapted in kind and proportion to constructive need. And, when the latter is satisfied, the hunger sense is quiescent, to return only when the organism again signifies renewed desire.

With the return of natural hunger after a fast, the food selective sensations, taste and smell, are discovered to be unusually keen and active. Too often are these faculties perverted by abuse to the extent of accepting and presumably enjoying food and odors that are abhorrent to naturally constituted organisms. At the conclusion of a fast, taste and smell act as co-indicators with hunger in determining the limit of abstinence; they, too, are restored to normal acuity. And with them thirst reverts to standard—not a desire for liquid that is produced by stimulation or by drug-exhaustion of the fluids of the body, but one that makes known the natural need for their replenishment. The being that eats when hunger, not appetite, calls, that drinks when thirst, not stimulation, demands, and that follows unquestioningly the selective sensations of taste and of smell, need never know disease.

It is sometimes good judgment to break a fast before the system is fully purified, then to return to abstinence after an interval of corrective diet. While this method is perhaps not as satisfactory in result as is that of the logically completed fast, it is at times expedient, and especially so in personally conducted essays into natural therapy, when there is lack of intelligent direction. Good judgment may also indicate shortening the period of abstinence when there is certainty of the presence of organic disease, or when preparation for the fast has been carelessly performed or entirely omitted. But, even though organic deficiency exists, the body is more certain of recovery when a fast is undertaken, since organic labor is thus gradually reduced, and progressive relief is afforded the system as a whole. In these conditions the sole hope either of partial recuperation or of ultimate cure lies in the systemic purification which the fast permits and in the rest afforded to the defective organ or organs which have been laboring under more than usual functional strain.

The question, "How long must I fast until my system is purified?" is one that may never be answered with certainty. Each individual develops his own case, and each case has its own limitations and requirements. And the further fact is to be faced that no matured human body in which disease is present may be brought to health within a definitely limited period of time. A lifetime of wrong living, more or less extended, has contributed to disease, and, especially in the chronic case, it is unreasonable to assume that nature, even when permitted a free hand, may within a few short weeks or months bring about the physiological changes necessary to function.

When a fast is successfully completed, the body functions in a sphere of natural activity, and no conception may be had, save in the indicated condition, of the gratification that accompanies the simpler acts that constitute physical life. To eat rationally, to eat only at the demand of hunger and not to excess, become pleasures that are exquisite, and that are not marred with regret for the flesh pots.

Nature asks of him who would live the balanced physical life but the will and the ability to follow logically the details of the simple law outlined in this chapter, the law of hunger, which, obeyed brings health for reward; but, which, violated, condemns the offender to condign and lasting punishment.

Breaking the Fast 11

Fruit Juices and Vegetable Broths: Gradual Return to Solid Food: What about Milk?

At one point in the discussion comment is made to the effect that one of the chief difficulties presented by the fast is its simplicity of application. In a sense this statement is paradoxical, but the method has been criticised adversely because of injudicious trial by subjects who deemed that the sole essential of this natural aid to health is abstinence from food. There are reasons that are obvious for this erroneous conception, which is based upon generally displayed and deplorable ignorance of the anatomy and physiology of the human body. Physical pleasure and physical pain are recognized sensations, but their causes, save as to the acts that produce them, are most infrequently investigated and are still more seldom understood, even when scientifically explained. The author believes that most mature intellects are capable of grasping the essentials of human anatomy and physiology, and for that matter those of any of the systems of therapeutics, that of medicine included.

But science has invented a language of its own—its terms are more or less foreign to the lay mind. And suffering humanity is not at all prone to devote many moments to the translation of prescriptions in order to discover the nature of their ingredients. What it wants is relief, and it wants it delivered with dispatch. And because humanity in general spends little time in educating itself in the care of its bodies, excepting in superficial ways, when illness occurs, it is necessarily dependent upon its physicians, to whose interest it is to offer to the patient assistance but not knowledge. It is really an attempt at release from this sort of dependency that causes the average mortal to grasp at some suggested remedy, whether it be a palliative that has relieved a suffering neighbor, or whether it be the promise of systemic purification which he is told will result from the omission of the ingestion of food for a time. But, again, in the average case, because of anatomical and physiological ignorance, difficulties are sure to arise. It is the desire of the author to present the details of the method described herein in statements so plain, so free from technical wording, that any seeker for truth in the cause of disease and its natural treatment may at once read and understand.

A fast should be undertaken only in the presence of disease, and it should be scientifically conducted. The latter statement should be taken as meaning that, in so far as the anatomical and physiological state of the patient may be discovered by symptom and examination, they should be observed and understood. Only in this manner may it be determined whether systemic purification by the interrupted fast or by one protracted to the return of natural hunger is the course to be pursued. If morbid conditions, other than those that are at first apparent, are latent, if the body has been carrying the burden of organs that are structurally defective, the fast is certain to uncover the facts, and it is then altogether probable that symptoms will develop that will need to be coped with by competent experienced hands. When, however, derangements that are purely functional are in question, a self-piloted case may progress to the end of the period of abstinence with success, but may not be able to solve the problem of breaking his fast assured of conserving all of its benefits.

An experienced director of the method is well aware that there are subjects, in number sufficient to be distinguished as a class, who, through physical defect in organs, store within the system food-poison in amount greatly in excess of that which is discovered in ordinary cases of functional disease. These subjects are to be grouped under Class 2 in the division of general disease forms tabulated previously. In them, constant stimulation, which is directly due to cumulative poisoning in progress, prevents recognition of the presence of the toxins themselves until some more serious indiscretion completes the overturn of physical balance. If now a fast is begun without preparation, difficulties are immediately encountered, for elimination commences with a rush of impurities seeking escape from the system, and, for a time, the tide is irresistible. Food cannot be taken, even though the will to eat exists, and abstinence must continue until systemic purification is accomplished. In these circumstances, during the first days of fasting distressing symptoms may develop, and dread of the outcome may lead to an attempt to supply food. If this is done, the trouble will be aggravated, for the whole organism is saturated with toxic material, and nourishment added then is just so much poison the more. Fear now takes full possession of family and friends, and perhaps of the patient as well, and the deadliest foe to the means that nature employs in dealing with disease is called to offset the work already accomplished. Medicine and neglect of the enema will then no doubt complete what food occasioned, and the chances are that death will ensue. In an instance such as this no defense of the method is accepted, and it is visited with widespread and emphatic condemnation; whereas, were the conditions observed received at their real worth, they would be recognized as natural and salutary in origin and action, and as evidences that extreme and successful organic effort towards cure was at work.

To break a fast in the manner described is a much more serious matter than to do so upon an incorrect dietary at the logical end of abstinence. But the point of greatest import here to be given attention is that of the confidence that should be engendered and the care that should be taken lest, when distressing symptoms occur, fear step in and with it food and drugs. Relief for localized pain and distress lies in the administration of copious enemata, duplicated and reduplicated, for only in this manner may prompt removal of their toxic causation be effected.

In the ordinary instance a successfully completed fast should be broken by the ingestion of the juices of ripe fruit or of broths prepared from vegetables. The juices of fruits that are fully ripened are most easily changed in mouth and stomach for subsequent digestive processes, and there is but small effort in handling them. The same reasoning is applicable to the use of vegetable broths, strained through a coarse kitchen sieve so as to remove fibrous material and hard solid particles. There are many vegetables that lend themselves readily to the preparation of these broths, and, when the latter are made as indicated so as to exclude all but finely comminuted solid matter, they are easily digested and their products are assimilated promptly and without difficulty. When using the juices of fruit to break a fast, it is suggested that those of sweet fruit be not mixed with those of acid. One fruit at a time is the rule. At first the broths should be confined in preparation to one vegetable, such as the tomato or the onion. Later they may be varied in ingredients, and combinations may be made of two or three kinds. The tomato is perhaps the one vegetable that lends itself most satisfactorily to the breaking of a fast, and it is in constant use for this purpose by the author.

As gradual approach to abstinence has been shown

to be conducive to success in outcome, so, after systemic cleansing has been wholly or in part accomplished, return to solid food should be brought about by degrees. The digestive organs have been deprived for a time of the exercise of their tasks, and, if at first overloaded and hence over-stimulated by surfeit, they are apt to refuse function, and toxication will perhaps recur with results that may prove troublesome. Hence it is recommended that, for several days after a fast is broken, not more than two pints of the broths described daily ingested, increasing this amount to three pints when digestion is fully reestablished. Vegetables in solid form may then be substituted, with, as a variant, salads of lettuce, tomatoes, and other like food-stuffs, alone or in combination. It is further recommended that a daily two-meal plan be thereafter adopted and adhered to, for, in most instances, with proper selection, two meals each day are ample for constructive demand. When return has been made to solid food after a fast, the morning meal may be confined solely to fruit, while the second repast should include a salad in some form or other.

In resuming feeding after fasting very young children it is found that the strained juice of ripe tomatoes, heated to about 200 degrees, or that of carrots boiled to tenderness, gives satisfactory results. Malted milk or orange juice and honey may also be used.

In some of the treatises upon fasting for the relief of disease patients are advised, upon the return of hunger, to resume feeding upon a dietary composed exclusively of the milk of the cow, gradually increasing the amount ingested until as many as eight quarts daily are consumed. The author differs widely from this recommendation, and reasons in support of this difference of opinion are here presented.

With slight variations referable to man the milk of the cow contains all of the nutritive compounds required by a growing animal, and it contains them in the proportions of a correct scientific dietary. Popularly milk is regarded as a beverage rather than, as in truth it is a nutrient vehicle most concentrated in the combination of its elements. In order to present a comprehensive idea of its composition, it is well to study the solid products of milk as they are obtained by various processes in the dairy, the kitchen, and the laboratory. It may also prove helpful to enumerate and describe the classes into which the solids of milk are divided. These are: (1) proteid; (2) fat; (3) sugar; and (4) mineral matter.

Fat constitutes about four per cent of the weight of milk. In the common process of making butter the greater portion of the fat is separated from the other ingredients. The liquid which remains, called buttermilk, contains the rest of the nutrients of the milk excepting those small portions that cling to the fat. On examining buttermilk after it has become a little sour, it will be seen that it contains a white solid which in the process of churning has been divided into very small particles. This solid is casein, the chief proteid of milk. It constitutes 3.3 per cent, or about one-thirtieth, of the weight of the milk

The souring of whole milk also helps to an understanding of its composition. When this takes place the casein and most of the fat separate from the still liquid portion (the whey), and form what is known as the curd. When, however, the attempt is made to separate the curd completely for the purpose of making what is known as cottage cheese, much of the fat is usually carried off with the whey. And again in the processes of manufacture of butter and cheese one becomes familiar with the solid, casein, and with the fat of milk. But even the whey, the liquid portion, has important solids in it that are less apparent and consequently not as well known. By heating whey it is discovered that it is filled with small particles of white matter that soon sink to the bottom of the liquid. This is albumen, a substance always present in cow's milk, though in much smaller amount than is the casein. It resembles the albumen of the white of egg, and it differs from casein by not curding when milk sours, and by remaining in solution in the whey. Furthermore it does not form curd in the stomach, which the casein does. This proteid which by the process of heating is shown to be present in the whey is the chief proteid in mother's milk, but in cow's milk it is, as has been said, in very much smaller amount than the curding proteid. Therefore, cow's milk, even if diluted and modified, can never be a perfect equivalent for human milk, and it is easy to understand that a proteid that remains dissolved in the whey is more readily digested than one which curds soon after reaching the stomach.

Milk also contains five per cent of sugar. This sugar is not like that which is used on the table, but is much less sweet, and it acts differently from ordinary sugar in the processes of digestion.

The mineral matter in milk constitutes about seven-tenths of one per cent of its weight, and it is more abundant in comparison with other nutrients than in any other common food. This is as it should be, for this material is in greater part intended for bone-building in the body of the calf. When taken into the human system, the amount of mineral matter present in cow's milk is much in excess of that needed for growth and repair, and, entering the circulation and not being available for constructive metabolism, it, like any other foreign matter, acts harmfully upon the organism.

Milk as secreted by the cow, and consumed as intended by the calf from its teats, is a food that is anti-acid in digestive reaction, but, delivered for human domestic use hours old, it is placed by fermentative changes in the acid-forming class. At the end of a short fast, almost without exception, the animal organism is in a condition of high acidity. It does not need a mind professionally trained to conceive of the result of pouring into a system in this state large amounts of protein, carbohydrates, and fat, especially in the concentrated form in which these elements occur in cow's milk. Nor is much mental effort required to comprehend the difficulties that are encountered by the eliminative organs in the attempt to rid the organism of its surfeit of waste, while both assimilative organs and circulation are forced to function with putrefaction at work at the source of supply.

Now there are cases which, after a fast, seemingly improve upon a diet of milk, but observation leads to the conviction that the benefits noted, if any, are due first, to the fast with its purifying effects, partial though they may be; second, to the one-food regimen imposed; and third, to the physical rest insisted upon. But whatever benefits accrue are in most instances temporary, and it is but natural that this should be so, for, even when the milk is handled without immediate distress, all of the organs involved in body metabolism are called upon to work to a degree that their labors are most inefficiently performed, and the possibility exists that they may break with the effort. It will be discovered that within a short time after the regimen described has been imposed upon a patient, the latter will have developed extreme congestion of the liver, high-colored, waste-laden urine, and systemic bilious saturation. And these cases always prove most difficult to bring to a purified state because of the toxic impregnation that follows milk-flooding.

In the present discussion the digestive capability under contemplation is that of a subject who has just succeeded in ridding his system in whole or in part of the toxic products of ingestion in excess of the needs of his body. In a partial fast it is deemed best to resume feeding, while in a completed fast hunger has returned and food must be supplied. If the milk of the cow is the form in which nourishment is offered, and if, in addition, not a small quantity, but, as advised, from four to eight quarts daily are imbibed, for each quart consumed, an equivalent in flesh food of about one pound is presented for digestion. The purpose of the fast is at once defeated, since the most vigorous of bodies is unable to transform and to assimilate this mass of material, however digestible it may in essence be. The excess, and it is virtually all excess, fills the alimentary tract with decomposing waste, and the system is again in the developing process of disease. And after all, the milk of the cow is intended only as food for the calf.

There are instances upon breaking a fast when some form of milk will be accepted by the digestive processes of certain individuals when those foods already indicated as suitable for the resumption of feeding are merely tolerated. In circumstances like these the milk of the goat is recommended for consumption, but in small amounts. Goat's milk in composition carries with it lesser quantities of mineral salts than does cow's milk it curds, not in masses, but in more or less separated particles when it meets the gastric juices while its fats are held in suspension, thus making them more easy of digestion. And there is this added advantage that the goat is not susceptible to tubercular infection.

When, after a fast, digestive power asserts itself, and the bowels begin naturally to respond, the enemata are gradually discontinued. Suggestions as to their use in health are given in the chapter devoted to a discussion of the internal bath, but it may here be said that natural movements of the bowels are dependent upon normal digestion; and this truth is but slightly qualified by saying that for normal function muscular tone is also a necessary condition in intestinal walls. For the attainment of the latter and for the rebuilding of general muscular quality, a system of exercise is recommended and insisted upon from the time that the fast is broken. This, like the dietetic regimen, should be entered upon in gradual manner, and should be increased and extended in proportion as the body shows progressive capability.

The procedure to be followed in breaking a fast demands both caution and care. At the end of a successfully completed period of abstinence, with hunger in evidence, weak-willed patients are almost certain to overstep the salutary limit of ingestion. In cases like these acute crises may develop because of congestion of the circulatory system. All of the organs of the body will be included in the revolt and the brain itself may suffer. When a gradual process of return to normal supply of sustenance is not pursued, the benefits of a fast are largely annulled; hence, if will power be lacking in the subject, its equivalent in supervision must be furnished by the director of treatment, and, if needful, personal watch should be established.

When there are structural organic defects in the colon, they may or may not prove shortening to life; but, when, at the end of a fast, feeding is resumed, even slight displacement in this organ may retard elimination to such degree that absorption of toxins will cause severe physical and even mental distress. This is especially liable to occur in those cases that are without guidance, in whom ignorance of the consequences of succumbing to desire exists, and will control is feeble. And, even under supervision, oftentimes, when desire impels and opportunity occurs, the patient will overeat. This tendency must be controlled, for serious results wait upon premature excessive demand upon the functions. Defective or normal in vital parts, man here learns to live within the limitations of his organs. Preparation for a fast, and the fast itself, are seen to be comparatively easy in accomplishment, but resumption of feeding after abstinence is a more difficult procedure.

12 Hygienic Accessories of the Fast

Breathing:
Bathing:
Sleep:
Exercise

BREATHING.—Nature has provided in the air that surrounds the earth a plentiful supply of oxygen, a gas that is essential to the maintenance of human life. Its function within the human body lies in replacing carbonic acid, a poisonous gas developed by the breaking down of tissue, and delivered to the lungs in venous blood. The interchange of carbonic acid and oxygen occurs in the lungs, since in the process of breathing, as carbonic acid is exhaled, oxygen is inhaled. The act of respiration exposes the blood, held within the thin walls of the pulmonary capillaries, to the air, and by mutual diffusion the two operations of oxygenation and of decarbonization are accomplished at one and the same time. The muscular movements made in breathing are not dependent upon the will, as this process goes in in sleep and in other unconscious states. The rate of respiration in health varies from fourteen to eighteen breaths per minute, and, besides carbonic acid, watery vapor and a small amount of organic matter are exhaled.

In order to furnish oxygen to the system, from three hundred to four hundred cubic feet of air are drawn into the lungs in twenty-four hours. Each hour an adult inhales about five hundred grains of oxygen and emits about six hundred grains of carbonic acid, with a much larger amount of watery vapor. Deprived of air, the body quickly perishes from asphyxiation.

Not only is a continued supply of pure air essential to life, but constant care is necessary to insure its purity at the moment of intake. The natural passages that carry air to the lungs begin at the nostrils, and these are furnished with short, fine hairs and with mucus secretion, preventives of the inhalation of dust and light material. If obstruction of the nasal tract occurs, it is possible for breathing to take place through the mouth, but so harmful is the latter method to general health that attention is here directed to its results.

A child that is overfed invariably develops a cold with accompanying nasal discharge and consequent obstruction of the natural air passages. A prolonged cold, or a series of colds, compels the use of the mouth for the act of breathing, a method that, if not corrected, eventually becomes habitual. Constant irritation and inflammation of the mucus membrane of the nostrils and of the vault of the pharynx cause the much discussed adenoid growths to form, and complete or partial obstruction of the air canal is thereafter permanent until removal of the obstacles is accomplished. In the ordinary manner this is done by the knife of the surgeon, but the shock to the organism of the child, both of the anesthetic and of the operation, is often productive of sequelae that persist through life, and this method for the removal of adenoid growth, so prevalent in recent years, is to be disparaged. In infancy and adolescence these annoying gland-like enlargements may not only be prevented in formation but may be removed through natural absorptive means, if proper attention is given to diet, and if short fasts are intermittently performed. In training the child in the care of his body, it is quite important that he be taught to free the nasal passages from gathered mucus at the least sensation of obstructive fullness. This is usually effectively accomplished by blowing the nose.

Children who are affected with nasal obstruction are more or less stupid and sluggish, and they oftentimes exhibit a facial expression approaching that of imbecility. In fact, when the habit of mouth breathing has been contracted, even when no obstacle is present in the naso-pharyngeal vault, not only do the nasal passages, through lack of exercise, fail of normal development, but the open mouth and dull eyes denote a serious deficiency in intellectual advance and capability.

We cannot know the exact source whence is received the influx of energy, the expression of which in the human body is life; nor are we yet aware of the manner in which vital force penetrates the organism and governs its movements and its thought. But life is evidently not inherent in the body, and, whatever its source, vital power must reach its vehicle of expression through surrounding atmosphere, through the air that the body breathes. Transference to the brain directly through the bony structure lying immediately above and back of the nasal passages is conceivable; and, while the purity of the atmospheric constituents that furnish the lungs with blood-regenerating matter may well be vitiated by transmission through paths not naturally intended, the lack of intellectuality of most mouth breathers cannot be accounted for on this basis. And yet it exists. Hence the theory here presented—that vital force enters the body from without through the natural air passages, passing to the brain through the bony cavities immediately above and in their rear. Whatever the attitude of the reader in respect to this thought, which holds place only as theory in the mind of the author, there can be no question of the importance to be attached to the cultivation of a nasal breathing habit, a habit that is at once preventive of disease and preservative of health.

In the fast correct respiratory methods must be pursued, and deep breathing is also recommended. Every portion of the lung surface should be exposed at all times to the general purifying process resultant from oxygenation of the blood, and to insure this contact, in addition to lung exercise, the body should be surrounded by fresh pure air day and night. Well ventilated living and sleeping rooms are important to the highest degree in illness and in health.

BATHING.—The skin or covering of the human body consists of an outer layer called the cuticle, and of an inner one, the corium. These constitute the true skin, but under them lies a third layer of cellular tissue, which is considered also as part of the skin, when that term is used in its most comprehensive sense. In man the skin is covered more or less with scattered hairs, profuse in some parts and scanty in others. The office of the skin is one of protection to the organs beneath, and it is also a vast excretory or eliminative system, sending out moisture with waste matter in solution through the sudoriferous or sweat glands located in its structure. Each of these glands consists of a long line tube, situated in the cutaneous cellular tissue and coiled into a knot near its closed end. This constitutes the gland proper. Then there is connected with it a straight or spiral duct that traverses the outer layers and ends in a surface opening called a pore. Nearly three thousand of the latter are found upon a square inch of the palm of the hand, and at least five-hundred on an equal space upon other parts of the body.

Perspiration is the watery matter "breathed out" from the system through the pores described. It is more copious than the exudation from the lungs by respiration, but the amount discharged varies greatly, as it is affected the heat or the dryness of the atmosphere, by liquids consumed, by exercise, and by the relative activity of the kidneys. Sensible perspiration is that which is perceptible in the form of small drops, but by far the larger portion exuded is of the insensible or non-visible kind. Solid matter is carried to the surface of the skin in the sweat, and authorities all agree that a considerable proportion of the total waste of the body is evacuated in this manner.

Close sympathy exists between the functions of the skin and those of the lungs, the kidneys, the liver, and the bowels, and this is evidenced in that, when one or other of the latter organs is disabled in function, perspiration is sympathetically deranged and vice versa. This does not necessarily mean that the effect produced is that of physical transference of the suppressed exhalation to the internal organ or the reverse, although this may be so; but the chief impression seems to be made upon the nervous system. The importance of the relation existing between the skin and the other excretory organs is such that it cannot be disregarded when disease is to be remedied.

In order to insure full functional activity of the surface of the body, frequent bathing is necessary. For this purpose one daily cleansing bath is essential in health. By it, dead, scaly particles of skin, dirt, and the products of perspiration are removed, the pores are cleared of surface obstruction, and the other eliminative organs are relieved of the performance of extra labor. When, as in the fast, the process of elimination is active in the extreme, cleansing baths may never be neglected.

A cleansing bath is a hot bath. One at temperature of about 105 degrees Fahrenheit is cleansing in the highest degree if pure vegetable oil soap be freely-used and the brush or cloth be vigorously plied. During a fast the temperature of the water in the daily bath or baths should upon entrance be approximately 100 degrees, and it should be gradually increased to as high as 107 or 110 degrees, with about twenty minutes submergence as the time limit. Baths such as this are not only cleansing, but are relaxing and tonic in effect. In cases of lowered temperature, habitual or temporary, the latter as in fasters' chilliness, correction to normal register, with systemic equalization of circulation, is rapidly effected by resorting to this therapeutic agency. Its very apparent benefits are due not only to the artificial raising of body heat, but to the process of osmosis, or interchange of fluids, that takes place in the capillary tubes constituting the pores of the skin. Cold baths should never be employed during a fast. They have but slight cleansing properties, but in health they exert a powerful stimulating action on the circulation and the nervous system.

Because of the oily nature of the waste brought by perspiration through the pores to the surface of the body, the skin can never be rendered perfectly clean with water alone. Hence the recommendation concerning the use of pure vegetable oil soap.

While the ancients made use of and elaborated the bath for purposes not only of cleanliness but also of social and intellectual objects, after the advent of Christianity and its domination of the civilized world, the bath fell into disrepute. Departure from the cleanly habit of body characteristic of early civilization was due directly to the rise and growth of the religion of Christ. The church frowned upon the care of the body, deeming it as negligible in comparison with the soul. And the early fathers in instances went so far as to impose penance upon those who gazed at the nakedness of their own bodies. Cultivated modesty, prudishness, thus had its part in the reversion that took place from the bathing habits of the Greeks and the Romans. Centuries later John Wesley uttered the aphorism, "Cleanliness is next to Godliness," but whether his reference was to the mind rather than to the body, it is impossible now to know.

Not so long ago the bathtub was generally condemned by medical authority in the United States, and about the time this was happening the cultured city of Boston by ordinance made bathing unlawful, save on the advice of a physician. However, be it said in extenuation of the hygienic condition of the Bostonese, the ordinance was characterized by slack enforcement and was finally repealed, but not until 1862. The good doctors of that generation averred that bathing, especially in winter, led to phthisis, rheumatic fevers, inflammation of the lungs, and to the whole category of zymotic disease. In the public prints bathing was inveighed against as subversive of democratic simplicity and of pioneer hardihood. And even today the medical profession is chary of advice regarding the hot cleansing bath, as, they say, it is weakening in its effects.

It is said that the first bathtub to be built and used in the Republic was that of one Adam Thompson, a citizen of Cincinnati, who installed his lead-lined, mahogany-covered receptacle in the year 1842. Water was supplied from the kitchen stove by way of the tea-kettle. His temerity appeared as a gross misdemeanor in the eyes of the press, the public, the medical profession, and the legislatures of those days. Later, in 1851, President Fillmore braved public opinion and placed the first bathtub in the White House.

There is no doubt that today in the mechanical conveniences connected with the bath, America surpasses the bathing arrangements of other ages and other races, but socially and sanitarily we have yet some distance to go before reaching the bathing standards and faciiities of ancient Persia, of Rome, and of present-day Japan. The ages-old warm bath habit of the Japanese causes them to look with the scorn of the elect upon those who are so uncivilized as to omit a daily hot cleansing bath. Yet it is this habit that is one of the great factors in that over-crowded land that makes for the remarkable health and vigor of the Japanese as a race.

The skin is the natural clothing of the body. Its protection to the parts beneath is aided by sub-cutaneous deposits of fat, a non-conductor of heat, distributed more or less uniformly over the body. When heated, evaporation of perspiration cools; when chilled, closed pores retain the body warmth. Like the lungs the skin permits of blood oxygenation through the walls of the capillaries, those small veins that ramify its substance, and, as has been stated, it is an organ of elimination as well. In the conservation of body heat, the skin is thermostat of the organism. It regulates temperature, and acts as a governor of internal function. If its work be interfered with by the interposition of substances between it and outer air, evaporation from its surface cannot take place freely, and elimination of the products of the pores is impeded if not arrested. In the latter case temperature is heightened artificially and abnormally, for prevention of skin activity causes retention of heat developed internally, and health suffers.

A striking exemplification of the close sympathy noted as existing between the functions of the skin and those of the other eliminative organs is given in cases of cutaneous burns where large areas are affected. Respiration is increased to exhaustion, and kidney discharges are heavily laden with waste that in the ordinary instance is eliminated through the pores. If an extreme proportion of skin area is seared, virtual suffocation ensues. Fatal results accompanied with symptoms similar to those in asphyxiation also follow when the body is covered with a substance, such as goldleaf, that is impervious to air.

In this connection it is not generally known that burns or scalds upon the skin may be successfully treated by submergence of the part affected in water. The exquisite pain of such injury is at once relieved by this procedure, and continuing the latter for hours or even days permits natural healing processes to act with dispatch and surety. If the skin area seared is extensive, placing the sufferer in a full bath and keeping him there for the time necessary will often serve to save life. The water in the tub should be at constant temperature and must be frequently changed, while water in quantity should be given the patient to drink.

The customs entailed by civilization are responsible for a number of physiological evils. While modesty is, in its origin, independent of clothing, for nakedness of body by no means involves the absence of this quality, nevertheless in civilized communities the world over modesty compels body concealment, and, because of conventional covering, the skin has for ages been permitted but partial function. Since clothing is deemed essential to decency, in order to reduce its effects upon the skin to a minimum, it should be fashioned of material as light and as pervious to air as is possible, while the skin itself should be cleansed and cared for with constancy and diligence.

Because of clothing the two great mediums through which energy is delivered to the human organism, pure air and sunshine, are in large part denied contact with its outer covering Clothing prevents full elimination of perspiration and its products, the latter remaining to clog the pores. This condition may be relieved to a degree by daily exposing the naked body to the air and to the light of the sun, and air-baths and sunbaths will be found valuable agents in compelling the skin to functional activity. During a fast, weather permitting, these baths should be taken with the subject upon the ground in open air.

In health a cold bath should never be undertaken immediately after a meal, but, with regard to a hot bath this caution is unnecessary. When the menstrual flow in woman is in progress, medical dicta to the contrary, a hot body bath and vaginal douche are daily essential for cleanliness and for relief and ease in function. The relaxing effect of a hot tub bath, together with resulting equalization of circulation, alleviates congestion and pain, if present, and in conjunction with other natural agencies cited herein, leads ultimately to permanent relief.

During a fast or while on restricted diet, the patient frequently experiences a sensation of chilliness with or without change in pulse and temperature. The source of this phenomenon, "fasters' chilliness," lies in nervous reaction following the absence of food stimulation, and, at times, in the absorption of liquid waste from the intestines. The enema will correct the latter condition, and a therapeutic bath taken as soon as the sensation of chill occurs will serve at once to equalize the circulation and to restore temperature and pulse to normal, if the latter are in any degree deranged. Baths for this purpose may and should be repeated as often as needful, if proper precaution is observed. In cases of greatly lowered vitality, when temperature is habitually below register, hot therapeutic baths should frequently be given, three or four daily usually proving not too many. Cold therapeutic baths for assistance in reducing fever should be more cautiously used. In any contingency, the therapeutic bath, hot or cold, should be administered only under competent direction.

SLEEP.—Sleep has its analogue in death; and it is an accepted scientific truth that the continuance of life in any living thing depends upon death. Through life to death; through death to life again. One manner of expressing this truth regards merely the outward fact, as when we say that animal tissue is renewed through decay; another regards the action and reaction proper to life itself, whereby it forever springs freshly from its source. And because of this inter-relation, this inter-dependency, between the two states of life and death, we apply to all manifest existence the term, Nature, which in derivation means "forever being born."

In the regularly recurring periods of unconsciousness, in the hours we spend in sleep, we find exemplification of the relation that exists between our working, active moments, and those that are devoted to the renewal of our physical and mental equipment. It is during sleep that the human instrument of thought and of motive government, the brain, obtains its repose; it is then that the cells of the human battery are recharged, that the working principle receives its potential for transformation during conscious intervals. It is then, too, that the greater portion of tissue impaired by wear in bodily activity is rebuilt and prepared for use in further exertion when consciousness recurs. Sleep is both a physiological and psychological necessity, and literal death will follow within short time if it be denied.

In the fast inability to sleep sometimes occurs, due in instances to lessened wear upon body tissue because of diminished call on muscles and organs, since muscular labor is more or less curtailed during abstinence from food, and digestion is entirely in abeyance. It may also happen that in the earlier stages of abstinence waste is excreted in amount incapable of being promptly and fully evacuated, and slight brain congestion with accompanying wakefulness results. The hot bath and the enema here again find their mission, and their use before retiring will go far towards remedying any tendency to insomnia.

But no natural process may be compelled if conditions be such that its function in the organism is not at the moment essential. Demand dependent upon necessity governs every natural desire. Upon it wait hunger, thirst, and sleep; without it, these constructive processes cannot be evoked. Hence frenzied attempts to induce sleep are futile, not to say foolish. The cultivation of an equable frame of mind in health, the ability to cast aside the cares of the day when one lies down to rest, add to disease-resistive qualities, and, if illness does occur, prove valuable aids to the efforts nature then proceeds to put into operation for relief. Here also reading plays its part; not that which necessitates extreme concentration of mind, but that which diverts the mentality, leading it along cheerful, wholesome lines of thought. The expedients suggested are natural abetters of healthful slumber, and find fitting time for their exercise after the activities of the day are done.

EXERCISE.—The maintenance of every muscle of the body in proportionate development is regulated by its work as well as by its supply of pabulum, although the latter is determined in large part by the necessity for repair or upbuilding occasioned by the exercise given the particular muscle. Constant use of one portion of the muscular fabric tends to add to its substance at the expense of that of neighboring parts not equally exercised. Hence the aim of all physical labor should be that of uniformity. Trunk and legs, arms and neck, all should receive proportioned attention. Normal muscular development also depends upon an unimpeded circulation of the blood and upon healthful cell-forming constituents uninterruptedly supplied for the replacement of used tissue. Constriction of the body in any region restricts free circulation, and only loose garments permit of full growth and proper development. The tight collar, the round garter, and the corset, make flabby muscles inevitable, and only a body unrestrained by the bonds so often prescribed by conventional usage can hope for muscular perfection. The possibilities of hygienic living, coupled with judicious exercise, are surely worth consideration, if merely for the satisfaction resulting from their effects upon personal appearance; but their more important consequences in respect to general health and longevity make neglect of these desiderata most deplorable.

Exercise that is self-imposed is wholesome; but exercise to which one is naturally attracted is the ideal form of labor. Combined with enthusiasm, physical work is doubly healthful, for enthusiasm in itself is a source of health. And that form of exercise that serves a productive purpose and is enthusiastically performed is best of all, whether the effort be physical or mental. Make your avocation the complement of your vocation. Gladstone and Horace Greeley chopped wood in their moments of relief from mental tasks. Conversely he who works with his hands should divert himself by exercising his brain.

During a fast moderate exercise in keeping with daily access of strength is advised, and, after the completion of the period of abstinence, constant comprehensive muscular activity is essential to tissue rebuilding and to form-development and maintenance. BR>

The Enema 13

Description of the Stomach and Intestines:
The Fallacy of "Purgatives":
The Principles and Use of the Edema:
Notes on giving the Enema to Children and On an Enema Tactic

The accompanying diagram of the human stomach and intestines is essential to a proper understanding of the digestive and eliminative functions of the body. It should be carefully studied in connection with the following description of the organs displayed.

"P. C.".—The Stomach.

This organ is a pear-shaped muscular bag, which receives the food after it has been masticated in the mouth. In mastication food is moistened and softened by the saliva, which also acts chemically upon certain elements, notably starch. Masticated food reaches the stomach through its upper or cardiac opening by means of a tube called the esophagus. Gastric juice, the normal secretion of the stomach, then begins its work of further transformation. While stomach digestion is proceeding, the liquid portion of the mass and the fluids drunk are in great part separated from the solids, and are at once absorbed into the circulation. The residue, called chyme, then passes through the lower or pylorio opening of the stomach into the small intestine.

"D. J. I."—The Small Intestine.

This portion of the digestive apparatus consists of a long tube, varying between twenty and thirty feet in length, which is ingeniously coiled upon itself. It is lined with what appears to be a soft velvety covering, an appearance that is caused by numerous minute elevations, the villi, which act as absorbents and secretents. In the upper part of the small intestine, chyme is subjected to the action of bile, the secretion of the liver, and to that of the pancreatic juice, the secretion of the pancreas, as well as to that of the secretion of the walls of the intestine itself. All of these juices still further soften and dissolve the food mass, and chemically transform the chyme into substances that permit of absorption through the villi into the blood. After the tissue-building portion is absorbed, the remainder—the refuse matter, the excrement—passes through a small opening known as the ileo-cecal valve into the large intestine or colon. This valve is constructed in such manner as to permit the waste to pass freely into the colon, but it prevents any backward movement or return to the small intestine.

"CC."—The Cecum.

The cecum is the large end of the colon situated just beyond the point at which the waste enters from the small intestine.

The Vermiform Appendix.

This is the small worm-like appendage to the cecum, which when inflamed gives rise to the trouble known as appendicitis. It is from one to five inches in length, and, despite the assumption that it is an organ that performs no necessary function in the economy of digestion, it finds its purpose and its use in adding stimulus, through its own motion and secretion, to the involuntary contractions and expansions of the colon, those vermicular movements called peristalsis.

"AC-R."—The Colon.

This organ, also known as the large intestine, consists of a tube about five feet in length, designated in the illustration as "AC", the ascending colon, "TC", the transverse colon, "DC", the descending colon, "SF", the sigmoid flexure, "R", the rectum at the extremity of which is the anus.

The colon is the main organ of elimination of the body, and through it the greater part of solid refuse is carried to the rectum to be discharged. When the colon is permitted to become clogged with food waste, the resulting condition is known as constipation, in which state fecal matter accumulates and renders the normally clean bowel a receptacle and retainer of foul, rotting refuse. The sigmoid flexure, "SF", is a device that prevents excessive pressure by the contents of the organ upon the muscles of the rectum, "R". Lying between the descending colon and the rectum it interrupts the straight fall from the transverse colon and it acts as a retaining pouch. The lower opening of the rectum, the anus, is guarded by a strong circular muscle which is under voluntary control.

The intestines as a whole are thus seen to consist of that part of the alimentary canal, which, commencing at the pyloric opening of the stomach, is coiled in the abdominal cavity and which ends at the anus. The several portions of the small intestine are known as the duodenum, the upper section, the jejunum, the middle section, and the ileum, the lower section. The lumen or tubular cavity of the small intestine is larger at its upper end, gradually narrowing as it goes downward.

The muscular coats of the intestines are circular and longitudinal in structure. In the colon the longitudinal fibres are proportionately longer than in the small intestine. Their greater length here permits of the formation of enlargements that often become the seats of fecal accumulation, and it is undoubtedly true that these cavities may contain fecal material that has been in process of gathering for weeks, months, or even years. Its presence and its products cause symptoms of disease to appear that vary from catarrhal inflammation to serious reflex disturbances. Excepting in extreme conditions, while quantities of waste may be held in these enlargements, a passage is necessarily maintained, and the main channel of the bowel still carries off feces. Occasionally a cavity becomes greatly distended with fecal matter, which hardens as its moisture is absorbed, and accumulations such as this have been mistaken for tumors or for malignant growths upon some abdominal organ. Impacted feces may occur in any part of the bowel, but chronic accumulations are discovered more often in the region of the cecum, in the ascending colon, and at or about the point of juncture of the ascending and transverse portions of the bowel, a condition that is to be expected, since in this part of the organ peristalsis works against gravity during the waking moments of the day.

Accumulations in the colon at times become so great that their weight tends to displace portions of the bowel, and several instances have been observed in whom the transverse colon from this cause had descended to the pelvis. In other cases the portion of the organ referred to, thus weighted for long periods, no longer lay normally just beneath the stomach, but occupied a position varying from slight downward displacement to a situation approximately in rear of the umbilicus. Fecal accumulations also vary in density, and they at times are so hard as to be mistaken for gall-stones. And again their mass may be so great as to press upon one or other of the abdominal organs, thus interfering with its functions. In this manner the liver is often compressed and its flow of bile obstructed, while the urinary organs may suffer likewise. In one observed instance, after thorough cleansing of the colon by means of an enema, a loss in weight of ten pounds was noted;

and in another fecal matter sufficient to fill a bedroom vessel of common size was taken from the bowel.

When feces are impacted in the colon it is difficult for the small intestine to perform its functions, for, not being able to discharge its waste freely, this organ in turn becomes clogged. Fermentation results, and the stomach is involved, while always the kidneys, the liver, the lungs, and the skin are forced to tasks beyond their capabilities, the two organs last named, in addition to their normal labor, being called upon to assist in the elimination of poisonous products not discharged, as they should be, through the bowels.

Fermentation and putrefaction of gathered waste in the colon at first occasion flatulent or gaseous distention, and the gas formed often encroaches upon the cavity of the chest, causing short and rapid breathing, and, when it invades the bend between the transverse and descending portions of the bowel, irregular heart action. As the result of pressure thus put upon the heart, death has often occurred, its cause being diagnosed as heart failure or organic heart disease. In other cases symptoms that have developed because of the formation of gas in the cecum and ascending colon have been diagnosed as appendicitis, and the patient has been operated upon surgically.

Long continued distention of the colon weakens its walls and causes the cavities or pockets already mentioned to form. Food not properly digested, not reduced to a condition adapted to the natural irritability of the intestines, may stimulate the colon to abnormal hasty contractions, as in diarrhoea, or it may prevent normal contraction of the organ. But, whether the fault lie in the quality of the food or in the digestive processes, the result is much the same. This observation applies as well to the ingestion of food in excess of the quantity needed for upbuilding and growth. In either case fecal matter accumulates because the colon is not normally excited to contraction, and cavities are formed because its fibres lose their natural resiliency from inaction and from the distention to which they are subjected.

It is of course to be understood that an impacted colon may result from a nerve supply insufficient to maintain the walls of the bowel in a state that will respond to the irritative presence of food waste. This constitutes a partial paralysis of the organ, and usually when inactivity of the kind is noted, it may in part be traced to spinal mal-adjustment or subluxation. In these circumstances the nerve fibres that transmit energy to the colon are impinged or pinched, and normal nerve vibration is prevented. In other words, motivating power is shut off at its source, and the sole means by which this deficiency may be corrected is by mechanical adjustment of the vertebrae involved.

A goodly portion of the information here recorded has been gained from examination of human bodies after death. In a number of these cases death was shown to have occurred because of ultimate organic inability of the intestines to function in that they had suffered in earlier years from lack of development, due either to insufficient nerve supply, the consequence of spinal malplacement, to bowel inflammation in infancy, or to the paralyzing influence of drugs administered for the suppression of symptoms.

In other instances of post mortem examination colons were discovered with walls lined to a depth of an inch or more with a viscous mucus-like deposit, portions of which must have been in process of collection for months. In fact, in several cases the entire length of the intestinal canal was thus affected. And, even when deficiency in development existed, impacted refuse was found in amount sufficient to occasion wonder that life in the circumstances could so long have been maintained, since in this condition only a minimum amount of food could have been digested, and the body had been supported mainly by liquids. Here the absorbents of the intestines were completely buried in the deposit and thus were rendered inactive.

In connection with the subject in hand the germ as a factor in decomposition occurring in the colon must be referred to. The large intestine in a general sense is to be regarded as a receptacle for body waste. It forms a suitable culture medium well supplied with warmth, and in conditions as we find them today, there are microorganisms constantly present that are capable of consuming toxic substances, and in their turn of producing them. When normal discharge of refuse occurs, the time of its retention is so short that the organ is comparatively free from soil in which microbic growth and propagation may proceed. Delay in evacuation gives time sufficient for germ development more or less extreme in character.

Ninety per cent of all drugs taken into the system under medical direction is aimed to affect the intestines. Evacuation of the colon, where there is constipation, is procured by the administration of a cathartic, a purgative. A purgative is a drug that is reputed to cleanse the bowels by frequent watery evacuations. But does it "cleanse" the bowels? The average conception of a cathartic is that it is a substance which through some power resident in itself removes fecal matter. This is not so. It moves nothing, either by mechanical or by chemical action. All cathartics, all purgatives, contain elements that are repugnant to both stomach and intestines, and that stimulate these organs into resistive action. In other words, they are poisons. When introduced into the system, they cause to be poured forth an augmented flow of intestinal secretion, which, to a degree liquifies the contents of the bowels, and, aided by similarly stimulated peristalsis, forces them to the rectum, thence to evacuation. The effect of the administration of a purgative then is one that results not because of any virtue peculiar to the medicine, but because the organs which it meets, objecting to the presence of a harmful intruder, act upon the drug and make instinctive efforts to cast it from the system. Any material introduced into the human body that cannot be utilized for its maintenance and growth is detrimental, and in a sense is a poison. This is true of all drugs.

Purgative medicines stimulate stomach and intestines to activities that are not natural, and they eventually bring about a refusal of these organs to perform their functions in a normal way. Once the purgative habit is acquired, the bowels after a time decline to act in the absence of the stimulus supplied by a pill or by some aperient. There is a homely saying that "castor oil loosens once and binds twice," and this is the very truth. Moreover the surfeit of digestive and other intestinal secretions called forth to expel the intruder causes the folds of the bowels to be filled with fluid fouled by dissolved waste, and the latter is partially absorbed ere evacuation can occur.

Extreme weakness results in many instances both from an unnatural drain upon these secretions and from poisoning of the circulation by absorption.

An apparently normal movement of the bowels may take place without clearing away impacted fecal matter. One may have a daily passage and yet be constipated. It is equally true that one may just have undergone a severe purge through the administration of a drug and still may have accumulation in the bowel. Nature at all times makes extreme effort to rid the colon of refuse, and in her striving a small channel is necessarily always open through the gut, else death would shortly occur.

If the taking of purgatives were confilled to adult life, the tale here told would be different in character, since functional derangement would be the principal harm effected. But cathartics are prescribed for infants and children in their growing years, and their indiscriminate use at this time of life is one of the great causes of intestinal non-development. Nutrition is lowered through digestive disturbance; inflammation caused by congestion is soothed by opiates; feeding and fermentation continue; development of the intestinal tract is arrested, or the tract in portions is paralyzed, thus affecting function. These conditions, if permitted to continue through adolescence, cannot be corrected by a lifetime of later natural existence.

It is evident that clean bowels are essential to perfect digestion, hence to pure blood, hence to health. The purgative fails in cleansing the colon. What, then, is the means to be employed when conditions such as have been described exist. When a conduit is badly incrusted with an accumulation of soluble matter, the course pursued to remove the coating is that of flushing repeatedly with clean water, and this is the process here advised when the colon is obstructed with body waste.

The enema, the internal bath, properly administered, will flush and cleanse the large intestine, will promote peristaltic action throughout the alimentary canal, and will fully suffuse the abdominal circulation with the most soothing and healthful of all fluids—pure water. And from its use there will result no depressing, no deleterious effects, either immediate or subsequent.

The enema or clyster has been known and used by

man for centuries. Herodotus, who lived and wrote five hundred years before the birth of Christ, says of the Egyptians: "For three successive days in each month they purge the body by means of emetics and clysters, which is done out of a regard for their health, since they have a persuasion that every disease to which men are liable is occasioned by the substances whereon they feed." However, the manner of administration of the enema then and thereafter was such as not to be as efficacious in result as we have later discovered it may be. The idea was held that an accumulation of feces had gathered in the rectum and in the folds of the sigmoid flexure. For the evacuation of this material a small amount of water injected into the rectum in a sitting posture was found to be easy and effective. This portion of the intestine may be cleansed by the injection of from one pint to one quart of water—in fact this is about its capacity, a larger quantity rising above the curve of the bend. It was also formerly doubted whether water could be forced above the flexure unless pressure was employed, and for a long time those who used the rectal bath made no attempt to cause the fluid to reach the descending colon for fear of injury. It has been demonstrated that the entire bowel can and often does become clogged and incrusted with refuse, and that larger amounts of water may easily and safely be injected into the organ flushing it throughout its length.

For the administration of the enema the sole equipment necessary is that of a fountain syringe with its rectal-tube attachment. The syringe should be suspended about five feet above the floor of the bath or lavatory, thus insuring sufficient fall for the water. Examination of the preceding diagram of the intestines will show that there are three positions in which the body may be placed in order that the colon may receive the water injected in such manner as to reach its entire surface, soften its contents, and wash them from its walls. These are the right-side, the knee-chest, and the flat-on-the-back postures. The last, excepting for children and for bedridden cases, is inconvenient to assume, but the two former positions are found to be comfortable and are easily taken.

When the subject in taking the injection lies on the left side, gravity assists the flow of the water only as far as the transverse colon, which in this position is perpendicular to the descending colon and forbids further passage of the fluid. Hence only the lower third of the bowel is affected. The right-side posture allows the water to flow along the descending colon, thence down the transverse colon and through the ascending gut to the cecum, thus completely flushing the organ. The knee-chest and the flat-on-the-back positions, obviously and with even greater ease, insure similar cleansing of the bowel. If, as is usual with those who are ignorant of the advantages of the postures described, the injection is administered while seated, gravity and the contents of the descending colon prevent the rise of the water unless some special device embodying force is utilized; and then again only the lower third of the bowel receives the benefit of the flow, and dilatation of the rectum and flexure is almost certain to occur with possible structural injury.

When a patient is bedridden or is extremely weakened, the knee-chest posture or the right-side position may prove too difficult or too exhausting to assume. In either of these contingencies, when no specially constructed table is at hand, a canvas stretcher upon which the subject may lie can be placed over the bath tub. If this apparatus cannot be procured, a triangular platform of three foot-wide boards covered with oiled cloth and a blanket, its base arranged so as to cross the top of the tub beneath the buttocks, may be used as a substitute. By the means indicated all effort in maintaining position is removed, a matter of importance in states of excessive weakness.

The operator in administering the enema, or the patient himself, in order to insure full benefit, will find it necessary to repeat the injection until the fluid returns comparatively colorless. This may mean that as many as twenty quarts of water may be required to obtain the desired result. Of course this amount of water cannot be introduced into the bowel at one time, but the contents of one bag or can, preferably of three-quart capacity, can be injected in the ordinary case and then evacuated with its accompanying refuse, and this operation may then thereafter be repeated until cleansing of the bowel is assured. Repetition as described is most essential in employing the internal bath, since the injection of only a small quantity of water acts detrimentally in that it serves to render the contents of the bowel readily absorptive, and is not in amount sufficient to be evacuated freely. Because of rapid absorption of the fouled fluid of the injection, retention of the water should be limited only to the time needful for injection and discharge. The latter may be facilitated by kneading the abdomen with the hands over the region traversed by the colon in the abdominal cavity.

Copious discharge from the bladder immediately after an internal bath is the common indication of the rapidity with which absorption takes place through the walls of the bowel, and it is seen that the process is almost instantaneous. For this reason salt, soap-suds, soda, and like substances should be avoided in preparing the fluid for injection. This caution likewise applies to the use of oil or glycerine. The only flushing agent should be water warmed to body temperature or not higher than one hundred degrees Fahrenheit.

When the enema is advised in medical practice as at times it is, invariably too small an amount of water is used, the posture is usually that of sitting, and, when what is known as a high enema is given, a colon tube, which is a long soft rubber hose, is attached to the fountain syringe. This accessory is not at any time needed, and its employment may prove harmful to the bowel. The short rectal-tube mentioned answers all purposes if the injection is taken in any one of the indicated effective positions. In any event the colon tube should be used only by an expert or under his direction.

Ignorance of procedure and erroneous reasoning have occasioned the belief that the use of the enema as recommended in the text will not only cause weakness in the patient, but will also bring about subsequent failure of function of the colon. It is contended that, once the enema is resorted to for any extended period such as is herein advised during a fast, natural movements of the bowels will not again occur, and that thereafter resort to the internal bath for colon evacuation will be compulsory. Natural movements of the bowels are directly dependent upon normal digestion, and in a system organically and functionally correct, peristalsis and subsequent discharge of refuse occur in sequence. In the course of the long experience of the author in the administration of the enema as described no instance of loss of bowel function nor of colon paralysis has ever occurred. On the contrary, the internal bath has been found to restore natural bowel action and to act as a tonic stimulus upon the muscles of the colon. Objection to the use of the enema advances as its basis the fact that for a day or so after full flushing of the colon no passage from the bowels occur. In the average case all bowel movements are evacuations forced by incoming waste from the small intestines pushing upon the contents of a filled colon, and the boasted daily movement actually consists only of discharge of the fecal matter contained in the rectum, the greater mass being still retained in the bowel. When, however, an enema has been correctly administered, the entire colon is cleansed, is emptied of its contents. The daily habit is consequently broken, and it may not be resumed for one day or several, or until the former condition of fullness has been restored which, if normal peristaltic function is impaired will shortly occur. Natural discharge from the bowels is assured only by attention to diet, to mastication, and to the existence of normal digestive processes, together with normal response of the colon to the irritative stimulus of waste deposited in it from the small intestines. And that man is the exception in whom this healthful sequence of function is the rule.

At times, even in those who have been accustomed to the use of the enema, difficulty is experienced in causing the water to penetrate beyond the sigmoid flexure. There may be slight griping pains when this occurs. Hindrance of the kind may be due to gas in the bowel or to nervous contraction of the muscles of rectum and flexure. If the difficulty persists, small amounts of water should be injected and discharged, this procedure to be repeated until the contraction ceases or the gas is discharged. Manipulation of the abdomen over the region occupied by the parts of the bowel involved usually affords prompt assistance, but, should the trouble prove obstinate, repeating itself at each attempt at injection, there is reason to believe that structural defect of some sort is present in the bowel.

In certain cases, when the enema is being employed daily under treatment, if there be in the subject a tendency to the formation of hemorrhoids or piles, these blood tumors may appear in and about the rectum and anus. In this contingency local application of some soothing emollient should be made to relieve irritation, and a properly constructed rectal dilator should be used to mitigate congestion. The symptom will not persist at length, and the enemas should continue notwithstanding slight inconvenience. But, while the hemorrhoids are in evidence, the dilator should be worn. It is to be borne in mind that in health the use of the internal bath twice weekly, as suggested herein, will preclude congestion of the rectum, and that hemorrhoids are unknown to one who employs this simple cleanly measure.

To revert to the condemnation visited upon the internal bath. Two cogent arguments lie behind this censure, of which one is commercial in character, for purgatives are sold at a price, and prescriptions also bring fees; the other is discovered in that an enema administered under medical direction is not correctly given either in posture or in quantity of fluid, and advice is usually proffered that the latter be retained for a time in the bowel. Hence these injections merely succeed in stirring up a filthy mass, putting it into condition to be easily absorbed, with increased auto-intoxication and subsequent depression as results. If a feeling of weakness occurs in a patient after an enema administered as described in the text, it is due to the removal of poisonous stimulation, the consequence of absorption from the contents of the colon. Once the accumulation is discharged and the bowel cleansed, recuperation is almost instant.

Physicians have also claimed that no appreciable

absorption of fecal matter in solution or of its products can take place from the large intestine. But medical science long since stultified itself in this respect when it recommended the employment of nutrient enemata in cases where feeding by way of mouth and stomach was refused. Denying that the contents of the bowel may be returned in part to the circulation through the walls of the gut, it nevertheless affirms that sustenance may in this manner be absorbed. It assumed and it still assumes that tissue may be nourished and that strength may be maintained by matter that does not undergo the process of normal digestion, introduced into the system by way of the colon. What occurs in this instance is stimulation, and poisonous stimulation at that, for material absorbed through the walls of the large intestine is received, not by the portal or nourishing portion of the circulation but directly by the venous blood, which already is laden with impurity awaiting oxygenation. Food substances introduced into the organism in this manner putrefy and poison. To deliver household water to the faucets through the sewers of a city would be deemed an act of insanity, yet analogy is plainly apparent when this method of transmission is compared with that of food injected into the body by way of the rectum.

In most cases during the development of disease the intestines are filled with food variously changed by the digestive processes but then in a state of fermentation; and the blood is laden with poison largely the product of morbific decomposition. The retention of excrement or waste in the alimentary canal, coupled with its disease-producing putrefaction, gives rise to bowel stoppage or constipation, and it may also cause the reverse condition, excessive liquid movements or diarrhea. Both of these phenomena are indicative of an unnatural, abnormal condition, are the immediate consequences of indigestion, and their toxic sequelae still further vitiate the entire organism.

Man in his natural state lived as nature dictated, and living naturally he was free from the harmful effects that arise from the retention of excrement in the colon, since fecal matter was not retained in the bowel long enough to be injurious. But man in his civilized state lives in many ways not naturally, and suffers in consequence. In natural conditions the human intestines are unobstructed by accumulation of refuse, and, as is the case with the lower animals, they are evacuated by frequent passages. This observation may be extended by stating the actuality that fecal matter in natural evacuations, refuse from the natural food of man, which was non-flesh in character, is almost without odor. That this is not true in the usual present-day instance needs no comment.

During a period of fasting the function of elimination is paramount, and waste from body tissue is cast into the intestines in profuse amount. The fluid state of this refuse permits of easy absorption, and its prompt discharge is imperative. From the beginning of abstinence until indications point to approaching completion of systemic cleansing, brownish, foul-smelling discharges are evacuated, and, in the earlier stages, hardened feces dislodged from the walls of the bowel are cast out in the enema. As purification progresses a feature more or less noticeable is the appearance of quantities of stringy white or yellowish mucus. This phenomenon is elsewhere commented upon, but the discharge is catarrhal in origin, although no inflammation of intestinal mucus membrane now exists. It consists of the remnants of impurity remaining in tissue structure, and is evidence of the complete purification that is accomplished by permitting the function of elimination full scope. Depending upon the responsiveness of the individual organism, this symptom is sometimes present from the beginning of a fast, and it is always noted in greater or less degree at some point during prolonged abstinence from food.

When fasting, the enema is an essential daily adjunct, and at this time it should be administered on rising, or shortly thereafter, and before retiring. In health, as a preventive of self-poisoning, an enema is advised at least twice in each week. It will be found a most relieving as well as cleansing operation, and it will obviate all chance of fecal accumulation, which means constipation with subsequent septic poisoning.

In a succeeding chapter mention is made of a procedure recently promulgated by both medicine and osteopathy—that of colonic therapy by means of what is known as cecal injection. This embodies the introduction into the bowel of a specially constructed colon tube of length sufficient to reach with its open tip the cecum. This being accomplished, the bowel discharge obtained, facilitated by injecting a solution of salt, is examined to determine the nature of the bacilli resident in the particular human subject at this point. These bacilli are then classified, and, if certain microbic forms are present, again through the colon tube an implantation by injection of bacillus acidophilus is made. The latter germ is said to have a very salutary effect upon the intestinal mucus membrane, and so to strengthen its powers of resistance as to cause it to withstand the attacks of any deleterious organism which happens to invade its precincts. It may be that the particular microbic infection of the cecal region is a mere amebic infestation—a simpler but more prevalent form of micro-organism than are those requiring to be confronted with a line of battle—and in this instance an antiseptic, consisting of kerosene and ichthyol, the latter a substance prepared from asphaltum, is forced to the domain of the enemy. This is followed by solutions of quinine, of emetine, a drug that has emetic properties, and of plain salt. No doubt the enemy at once retires when this onslaught on his forces occurs, but what of the poor victim whose body he inhabits?

No intelligent reader of these lines can fail to be impressed with the comparison between that method of therapy which insists upon attacking the outposts of disease, its symptoms and the regional abodes of its micro-organisms, and that system of healing which contends for the eradication of the cause underlying the existence of both symptom and bacilli. That the enema, administered as described in this chapter, in conjunction with the eliminative effects of the fast, does all that may be claimed for palliative, temporary agencies, one of whose tedious procedures is here detailed, is patent. And they accomplish much more, even to the ultimate desired result, bodily purification, rendering through their offices every organic secretion physiologic, hence resistive, rather than pathologic, with no power to repel organism inimical to health.

Note I

Details of administration of an enema to the infant.

The usual fountain syringe should be used, equipped with convenient length of tubing, with shut-off, and a small-sized rectal tip. An extra unattached tip should be at hand, the use of which is later explained.

There should also be a low chair or stool admitting of holding the recumbent child in the lap at a height slightly above the level of the bowl of the toilet.

Two pieces of rubber sheeting are needed, each one yard in length. One of these should be thrown over the top edge of the raised seat of the toilet, draping it so that it may receive spatterings and forcibly ejected discharges. The other should be placed one-half over the lap of the operator, permitting its free end to cover the front edge of the toilet bowl with sufficient length dropping over the inner edge to convey discharges into this receptacle. A folded Turkish towel should be laid over the end of the sheeting on the lap in such position as to be under the buttocks of the child, thus raising them slightly and preventing contact with the surface of the sheeting.

The operator should sit with right side next the toilet bowl, with the infant lying upon its back across the knees.

Care must be observed in inserting the rectal tip into the anus, and the right hand of the operator should hold it in position after insertion and while the water is flowing. Greasing the tip with olive oil or with an antiseptic lubricant will prevent irritation of the membrane of the orifice. The flow may be regulated by the shut-off or by pinching the soft rubber tubing with the thumb and forefinger of the left hand.

In small children during the administration of the contents of one bag of water, it is usually not necessary to remove the rectal tip from the anus, since the liquid form of the discharge permits ejection around the sides of the tip, and repeated insertion and withdrawal with possible chance of irritation is thus avoided. After the exhaustion of the water in the syringe, the attached tip should be withdrawn, and the unattached one mentioned as part of the equipment should be introduced into the anus. Through it evacuation of that portion of fluid retained in the colon will occur the more easily, since by this means constriction of the muscle of the anus is overcome. Neither pipe should be inserted to greater depth than two inches. At this stage of the procedure manipulation should be made of the abdomen, following the ascending colon on the right side from the cecum to the transverse bowel, thence over the transverse section to the descending colon, thence down the left side to a position corresponding with its extremity and outlet. This is an essential that should not be omitted, since it assists peristaltic action and hastens evacuation. The total quantity of water injected in giving this enema should not be less than six quarts, and, if extreme discoloration in discharge persists, more fluid should be used. It is of course understood that it is not possible to inject this amount of water into the colon at one time, but that repetition in injection and discharge of fluid is here implied.

Note II

Several positions are indicated as suitable and efficacious when an enema is administered, but perhaps that which will insure both comfort to the subject and complete flushing of the colon is the flat-on-the-back posture. In order that this may be conveniently assumed, a specially constructed table is of great assistance. A table, such as this, now in use at the sanitarium of the author, carries the following measurements: Length of top, over all, 44 inches;

Width of top, over all, 18-1/2 inches;
Height of rear and higher end, over all, 23-1/2 inches; Height of front and lower end, over all, 16 inches.
Four sturdy legs, properly braced, support the top.
Lengthwise from the middle of the top, grooves, such as are carved into drain boards, run to the lower or front end of the table, thus permitting surplus water to be guided to the receiving vessel, usually the bowl of the toilet.
A semi-circle of four and one-half inches' radius is cut into the center of the lower end of the board that forms the table top.
This stand should be placed in front of a toilet with its lower or front end projecting partly over the bowl.
The subject, with head supported by a small pillow lies upon the table on his back, with feet raised so as to rest upon the upper edge of a low toilet tank.
In order to guard against spatter from discharges, an oil cloth sheet should be draped over the front of the toilet tank, with its lower edges extending below and inside the roll of the bowl. This sheet should be attached to wall and end of table in any convenient manner.
Instead of the usual fountain syringe, the author employs a tank of galvanized iron, holding approximately four gallons of water. Its measurements and shape are as follows:
A flat back 10 inches wide by 15 inches high;
A semi-circular front, 19 inches around from edge to edge of back, to which it is soldered along the 15-inch edges;
A semi-circular bottom piece soldered to the two pieces already described;
Two stout metal lugs, holed for screws, are riveted to the top edge of the back for wall supports;
A substantial and convenient small faucet is soldered into the center of the lowest point of the circular front of the tank. To this faucet are attached five or six feet of rubber

tubing with the necessary rectal tube inserted at the extremity.

By the use of the table described the internal bath may be administered with but small effort or inconvenience either to patient or operator. In case of inability on the part of the patient to perform the acts necessary to the procedure involved, the operator should seat himself on the right side of the subject, in which position he can easily insert and extract the rectal tube, as well as control the flow of water into the colon.

This auxiliary appliance is of the greatest assistance in administering the enema to children, to the very ill, or to the helpless bedridden sufferer, and it is often preferred by those who are able to assume the various positions and to perform the necessary acts without the help of another.

The tank, for which measurements are given, is also a convenience, in that it obviates successive refilling of a rubber bag or hospital douche of small capacity. It should be suspended upon the bathroom wall with its bottom about five feet above the floor, this height giving through gravity just about the correct amount of force to the flow of water entering the bowel.

The author expresses the opinion that her experience in the administration of the internal bath is greater than that of any other known exponent. And out of that experience have evolved the two appliances here described. They have proved invaluable additions to comfort, cleanliness, and ease of performance in what is always an unpleasant but necessary task attached to the practice of natural therapy.

Note III

Those who do not wish to go to the trouble and expense of building their own apparatus, as described in Note II above, may find the J. B. L. Cascade an easy and convenient method of taking an internal bath. This device is distributed by Tyrrell's

Hygienic Institute of New York, and it may be found at most good drug stores carrying rubber goods. The author considers that, for taking an internal bath, the J. B. L. Cascade is the most effective and most reliable of the many patented devices that have been put on the market.

Children in the Fast 14

Various Errors Concerning the Care of Infants: Why Feed a Feverish Child?

When the human child is born into the world, it is equipped with but three developed faculties—hunger, thirst, and sleep. The infant, if capable of expressed desire, would signify its greatest need as sleep, but its rest is naturally punctuated with hunger periods, and at these times and at no others it should be fed. To awaken a quietly sleeping child for the purpose of administering food is most inadvisable, yet nurse and mother, burdened with professional tradition and advice, in over-zealous care rarely permit a two-hour interval to pass without forcing food upon the attention of the baby. The child will through habit take the breast or the bottle and suckle for a while, but its rest has been disturbed, and its small digestive apparatus is never free from labor as long as these misguided women can stimulate appetite. Disobedience to natural law brings its penalty, and disease shortly appears to right the wrong. Overfeeding a child is the greatest cause of infantile disease, and it could not occur if the first hunger instinct were permitted to guide the infant from birth. Actual need alone would then be satisfied, and the artificial sense of appetite that invariably develops when overfeeding is the rule would never appear.

Another error in connection with the earliest living moments of the infant is that of haste in severing the umbilical cord, the physical bond between the child and its mother, before the cessation of its natural pulsations. Interchange of oxygen and of nutriment between mother and fetus has taken place through this avenue during the whole period of gestation, and by this means the baby frame has been built to the moment of birth. Its final use and its last pulsations insure tissue nourishment sufficient to carry the child until food for post-natal growth can be furnished from the breast of the mother. Haste in cutting the cord starts the infant badly, and hunger is asserted much earlier than should be the case. In addition, babies thus treated often exhibit anemic tendencies because of mother-blood denied at birth, while their metabolism is compelled to function much too soon, and the mother herself suffers uterine and placental congestion with possible delay in the expulsion of the latter organ. It may be noted that undue retention of the placenta in whole or in part is the cause of death of thousands of women at child-birth or shortly thereafter.

When departure is made from the laws of nature, abnormal physical conditions are produced, and penalties are exacted. The normal food and the only food that is designed for infant use is mother's milk. At birth, delay in its appearance is often noted, and per-

alties are exacted. The normal food and the only food that is designed for infant use is mother's milk. At birth, delay in its appearance is often noted, and perhaps for two or three days its secretion is absent. Reference to the function performed by the umbilical cord before birth and at delivery offers explanation why in this event undue haste need not be made in attempting artificial feeding. If, as unfortunately is too often the case in modern life, the mother finds herself incapable of furnishing food for her child, a substitute must be obtained. The ideal method makes use of the wet-nurse, but, if this cannot be done, water-diluted full goat's milk, with sugar of milk or honey added, sufficient to supply as nearly as possible the constituents of mother's milk, is the nearest and best alternative. When the milk of the goat is unobtainable, top-milk from a healthy cow may be utilized. Prepared foods are doubtful in efficacy. There are many kinds on the market and the possibility exists that one or the other of these may agree with the particular infant. Orange juice and tomato juice are also additions that should enter the dietary of the child, supplying as they do vitamins and mineral salts, elements most essential to body maintenance and growth.

Whatever physical handicaps the mother may endure, the child in her womb receives from her body the best in the way of nourishment that that body is able to give. This is well exemplified in an earlier chapter when illustration was made of pregnant women, ill and fasting, who yet brought healthy children into the world. And, too, the contention that all disease has its origin in impaired digestive power is more strongly upheld when disturbances occur in the young than when adult organism is affected. In the child, unaccustomed to continued abuse of the body and its functions, and with no harmful habits formed, the system resents to its limit any but natural treatment. And it is especially during this period of early infancy that measures for the prevention of later disease should be first in the thought of the natural guardians of the child. Future physical welfare absolutely depends upon the running start which can then be given, and every source of information that offers logical guidance in hygiene should be exhausted, and the knowledge gained should be applied. Herein lies the extreme value that is to be put upon the principles exploited in the text. As against forced feeding, we have the natural instinct of the child, which, when normal, indicates its food requirements even to the point of partial selection. If by accident disease occurs, as against suppression of the symptom, we have the assistance offered by the fast and its eliminative aids to purify the system and to eradicate the cause. And this gained knowledge has the further worth of coming, not by hearsay, but straight from nature itself, by which token it is to be the more cherished and conserved.

The physical condition of a nursing mother is always reflected in the body of her child, and mental disturbances, temporary or permanent, show like effect. Through nervous derangement of functional power, induced by disease or by anxiety, grief, or anger, such changes are occasioned in the milk of the mother as to cause serious illness in the sucking child. It is therefore incumbent upon this parent so to regulate her physical body through a dietary regimen as to prevent error in milk quality, and so to conserve her mental forces as to prevent systemic poisoning through emotional tension, with their detrimental influences upon infant digestion.

When infantile disease is manifested, a medically treated child is still more hampered in its physical processes. Drugs are poisons, and their introduction into the body of an infant suffering from food excess or from the results of erroneous diet on the part of the mother, works havoc with tender nerves and tissue. Drugs aim at the suppression of symptom and not at removal of cause, and many an adult organism is compelled to struggle through life handicapped by undeveloped, partially paralyzed mechanism, the result of dosage in infancy.

The disease symptoms of childhood frequently assume epidemic form. Contagion and infection actively affect the individual only when his physical state is such as not to be able to repel the germ, either of the ever present variety or introduced from outside sources. The aim of the parent should be directed toward the preservation of health with its resistive qualities in the body of the growing child, and if, through carelessness or ignorance, or accident, this condition may fail of conservation, toward the prompt removal of the soil in which the germ thrives and dies. To use a germicide in these instances is suicidal, for germicides merely succeed in destroying the microbe, a process that adds decomposing material to an already fertile and expectant medium. And it is reasonable also to assume that a poison powerful enough to kill living organisms within the body is of strength sufficient to deal destruction to the cells composing it.

Referring to a former statement concerning feeding the body while high temperature prevails, the question may be asked:—Why put food into the stomach of a feverish infant! A roaring fire is not ordinarily subdued by adding fuel to the flame. Fever is in actuality a salutary symptom indicating by its very existence an active internal struggle by natural forces to rid the system through rapid combustion of material that is most inimical to life. It is caused by absorption into the circulation of the products of excess food rotting in the alimentary canal, and, when additional material is forced into this mass, the results are a further rise in temperature and added distress. Should drugs be administered, they are either stimulants or narcotics, the former increasing the action of the heart and with it the temperature, the latter reducing nerve sensibility and power. In the body of the child the effects both of overfeeding and of drugs are long-lasting, and here, as in all disease, the method to be employed should be that which will tend to remove the ferment, the rotting material, the cause of the condition.

Hence, as in the adult when illness appears, prompt

withholding of food permits of active elimination of the cause of disturbance; an enema or several of them cleanses the bowels of toxic substances; fever is at once abated; diarrhea and colic vanish; and in two or three days at most the youngster is again whole and hearty, ready for normal functioning. For children respond to the fasting treatment in marvelous manner; their natural forces have not been depleted by years of excess in physical indulgence, and are present in pristine vigor. And with them no argument is needed as to the efficacy of the means employed, for their mental habit is not as yet sufficiently molded to prove combative.

A fast until hunger makes its demand is mandatory in even the slightest digestive ailments of the smallest of babes; and a comparison of this method of treatment with that which requires the stomach to be dosed with drugs and the system to be permeated with the products of disease developed in the lower animals and introduced into human blood in the forms of virus and of serum needs no commentary excepting that of extreme condemnation for the latter procedure.

When the enema is administered to children an amount of water should be used that is commensurate to the size of the immature bowel. If the internal bath be thoroughly but judiciously employed, the colon of the child will be flushed of poisonous content, fever will subside, and disease will vanish. The enema may be given even to the day-old babe with beneficial results, for it serves to cleanse the colon of its pre-natal secretion, always productive of harm if retained. The ease with which a fretful; colicky child may be relieved by the careful use of the internal bath is a matter which every mother should understand, and the employment of the enema at judicious intervals during infancy is of equal importance with its use in adult life.

Whenever in a young child the smallest indication of disease appears, whether it be in the form of nasal discharge, of constipation, of diarrhea, or of internal pain, it should be considered as full warning of loss of balance between nutrition and elimination. Food should at once be withheld, the enema administered, and this form of treatment continued until equilibrium is restored. If the situation be handled thus, there will be no later development of acute disease; no adenoids, degenerated tonsils, nor other morbid organic structural defects will evolve. Care of this sort at this time precludes dependence upon the knife of the surgeon in infancy, in adolescence, and in adult existence. In other words, prevention through systemic purification is the greatest hygienic need at this age and at all ages, but it is the more essential in infancy, which is the physical and physiological formative period of human life.

Sexual Disease and the Fast

15

Menstrual Difficulties: The Menopause: The Orthodox and the Natural Approach to Gonorrhea and Syphilis: Masturbation

The ultimate of therapeutic fasting is accomplished by the restoration of all physiological function to normal, and, when success attends upon abstinence, normality is the rule, not only with respect to the processes of nutrition, but to those of the sex functions as well. In fact, the organs of sex respond perhaps more readily than do other vital parts to the restorative agencies invoked by reason of abstinence from food.

In woman during a fast the menses may or may not appear. If they do, usually before the period there is disturbance nervous in character, and the flow, either scanty or profuse, may be viscid in consistency and perhaps offensive in odor. After feeding is resumed the monthly discharge may miss one or several periods. Its absence should occasion no anxiety, for in a sense the menstrual flow is at all times a waste product, and in a successfully conducted and completed fast systemic purification has been achieved and but little refuse, if any, remains to be eliminated. Accumulation must again take place ore the periods may be reestablished.

With respect to the menstrual discharge the interesting facts are to be observed that it is of regular recurrence during the bearing period in the females of all mammals; that it is barely perceptible in some; and that in none is it so profuse in quantity as in woman. She is the only female in the animal kingdom who is compelled to undergo a monthly inconvenience of copious flow from the organs of sex. Yet this evidence of function, as natural as is breathing, because of perversion in habit has become aggravated in degree. Profuse discharge from the uterus is the penalty attached to the use of the organs of reproduction for purposes other than those that are legitimate—a perfect demonstration of the universal law of compensation.

In treating disease of the reproductive system in woman, the fast tends both to cleanse and relax, both to relieve congestion and to restore tone. From one to three days without food will serve, in conjunction with accompanying eliminative aids, to correct excessive menstruation, and, when no structural organic defect is present, relief is apparent within twenty-four hours when the flow is attended with pain. In this connection attention is directed to the use of the hot douche, the hot bath, and the enema at the time of the monthly period. It is difficult to assign adequate reason to the strong objection generally made by medical practitioners to the cleansing douche at any time, and especially to its employment when the menstrual flow is on. Cleanliness of the organs of sex is always imperative, and cleanliness with freedom from danger of infection cannot be attained during menstruation unless the parts are bathed both externally and internally. Medical opinion to the contrary, the hygienic accessories mentioned are at all times helpful, and are doubly so when the menses appear.

The menopause or change of life is dreaded by all women. There is never any certainty as to the time of its occurrence, nor any means of foretelling the character of its manifestations. As treatment by means of the fast demonstrates that the menses may be regulated and that assurance of their normal recurrence is possible when natural law is followed, so similarly purification of the system at the time of the menopause, or better, before its appearance, coupled with a correct dietary and judicious exercise, will permit any woman to pass through this experience without evil consequences.

At the time of the change of life many surgical operations are performed upon those women whose previous existence has been such as to foster functional sexual trouble to the degree that structural organic defect in sex organs develops. Then appear fibroid conditions in uterus, affections of various sorts in ovaries and fallopian tubes, and always vaginal discharge abnormal in character. It is useless at this time to indulge in regret because of bodily abuse in the past; the harm has been done; yet, in most instances, these conditions of disease may be remedied, and prevention of surgical operation may be assured by employing the agencies exploited in these chapters. And, previous to the menopause, unless congenital organic disease exists, so-called female troubles may successfully be combated, in fact, need never be known, if the dictates of natural law are accepted and obeyed.

Because of the prevalence of varied forms of sexual distress in woman, not only at the change of life, but throughout adult existence, the object of the fast and its natural eliminative accessories is again repeated and emphasized. At all times the end to be accomplished through abstinence from food is that of bodily purification, systemic cleansing. When correctly administered, a fast for therapeutic purposes causes allergic avenues to be cleared of obstruction, healthy tissue to be deposited in place of that which was diseased, and vital organs to be recuperated to the point of extreme ability to function. By virtue of these achievements the high office of reproduction in woman is not only healthfully stimulated, but is restored virtually to primal ease in gestation and in delivery of offspring. And, when the bearing period ends, the conditions of disease that are its usual accompaniments may, by the means described, be obviated, or, if present, may be relieved to the point of recovery and the enjoyment of future health.

In discussing the problem of sexual disorder of any

kind and its relief, but especially with reference to what is known as venereal disease, it is necessary to revert to the primary cause of illness of any sort, lowered nutrition resulting from impairment of the digestive processes. If the individual system be at high resistive level, if the products of elimination be normal in character and are promptly removed as they are produced, the bacillus of gonorrhea, for instance, transferred by contact to either sex, cannot find foothold for increase. It is only when the balance between nutrition and elimination is at fault, when physiological resistance is lowered through digestion defective in function, that infection may occur.

In the past, orthodox treatment of venereal disease has been responsible for much subsequent annoyance and distress, and present prevailing methods of handling this sort of illness show but small improvement over those of the past. Deep injections of antiseptic drugs, aimed at the suppression of nature's curative effort as exhibited in copious secretion issuing from mucus membrane, are always productive of increased irritation, and usually leave as sequels of a gonorrheal infection, gleet, urethral stricture, and prostatitis, if not worse, all more or less permanent physical injuries. Much more logical, and immeasurably more easy of application, are those means by which natural curative processes are assisted and accelerated. Omit food, ply the enema and the bath, rest, and the irritating symptoms will not only subside within a few days, but will disappear, to leave behind them no supervening ills.

And what is true of a symptom, which, like gonorrhea, is in a sense merely local in character, is equally true in the treatment of the dreaded blood taint, syphilis. Here again the criticism is offered that orthodox remedies administered for the suppression of syphilitic symptoms produce effects that are worse in comparison than those of the blood taint itself. Whether congenital or acquired, this symptom, if subjected to the purifying processes of the fast and its accompanying eliminative aids, before the organic lesions characteristic of its later stages develop, will yield to the treatment with success. There will naturally be more difficulty attendant upon its eradication from the system than is the case with gonorrheal infection, for syphilis is the more deeply seated symptom and affects the blood itself, hence it partakes of the nature of structural defect in a vital organ. But, if it be taken in time, through fasting, systemic purification will surely occur, and eradication of the syphilitic taint be accomplished.

Masturbation, like all other forms of perverted natural function, is of more widely common practice in both sexes than is generally believed. Its beginnings usually occur through the curiosity of pubescence, and it is further stimulated by vicious influences, if these are at hand. But its development into habitual excessive form requires constitutional derangement that combines both physiological and psychological causes in its evolution. A discussion of the latter cannot here be made, but in close connection with the subject matter of the text lies the truth that children fed upon a non-stimulating diet, one free from flesh and embodying only such amounts of the higher forms of protein as are needful for normal growth and bodily maintenance progress to puberty in gradual development, showing fewer tendencies towards sexual abuse or perversion than do those whose dietary includes the flesh of animals and other stimulative kinds of food. Yet, if the habit be developed, again the fast offers relief in the removal of the general cause underlying all symptoms of disease, with the restoration of a condition of morbidity to one of health.

Food and Disease 16

The Purpose of Food:

Why We Overeat:

Objections to the "Germ Theory":

Mucus Discharges

The processes by which dead food is transformed into living matter within the animal body are purely chemical in character, and, for the reason that these operations are accomplished involuntarily, they are in a sense mechanical. In essence the purpose that food serves in the organism is that of furnishing material for the rebuilding of cell structure when the latter has become exhausted by the destructive effect of work performed. The changes involved in the preparation of food for conversion into living tissue are sufficiently familiar to preclude description here. But the act of digestion involves an effort that is at once nervous and muscular, and in it energy is liberated, utilized, and dissipated, and, in so far as the expenditure of what may be called nervous force is compensated, a balance is maintained.

If, however, the process of digestion is permitted to proceed to a point beyond actual reconstructive need, chemical action and reaction are thrown out of poise, and the result is disease. And, too, when the system is surfeited with sustenance, energy that should be utilized for other important metabolic purposes is necessarily employed in the attempted disposal of matter in excess of what is needed for replacement of used tissue. Some of this material is absorbed by the assimilative processes, and surplus thus accumulates in circulation and in the cells of muscular and organic tissue. The liver, laboring to its functional limit, segregates and casts out what it can, and its largely increased bilious product, together with undigested matter in the intestinal tract, if not promptly evacuated, ferments, germ soil is provided, and absorption of toxins proceeding from active decomposition and from evolved bacteria occurs rapidly and continuously. Small wonder that, in the circumstances, natural avenues for the passage of energic force are clogged, that imperfect functioning occurs, and that disease follows!

Only that portion of digested food that is assimilated can be used for the repair of cell structure; the remainder is refuse that not only adds dead weight to the body, but that, in its disposal, vastly increases the labor of every vital organ. There succeeds a waste of energy that is shown in diminished digestive and assimilative power, with resultant lowered vitality. And any disturbance either of the function of digestion or of that of assimilation sends into the circulation blood-forming material that is elementally deficient, a condition that assures defective tissue nourishment.

A review of the physiology of the passage of the blood through the body evidences that health is synonymous with perfect blood quality and circulation. Given a pure blood supply properly delivered, the products of converted food are carried to their varied destinations, and cell waste is gathered and promptly eliminated. The maintenance and well-being of the animal body is directly dependent upon the normal performance of the process outlined.

An examination of human fecal discharges in the average instance reveals conditions that are conclusive. Undigested food is discovered, digested food products and old feces are present, and, dependent upon the dietetic regimen and the preliminary processes of digestion as carried out by the individual, the odor is more or less offensive. Normal refuse from properly masticated, correctly digested food, not animal in origin, is not disagreeable in odor. Again in the average case, when daily examination of bowel passages is continued for a time, assurance is gained that all ingested food is not digested; that the colon is not completely cleared of waste even by regular daily movements; and that fermenting matter defiles the interior to a degree scarcely to be accepted as a fact.

A movement of the bowels each day is never a certain indication of a clean and healthy alimentary canal. Sufferers from digestive troubles often assume that, because the bowels are regular in action, the evacuations must be complete and sufficient. This assumption presumes physiological ignorance, for in these subjects usually the rectum alone, daily filled with a mass of waste forced downward by that which is retained in the colon, is relieved of its contents. If, after such an evacuation, a full enema is administered, indubitable evidence of extreme internal filth will be produced. Post mortem dissection of the colon in the average cadaver but adds weight to the substance of the statements here made, for fecal matter of more or less remote production is discovered lodged in the sacculations of the organ and upon its walls. In these circumstances during life, a movement of the bowels takes place through the center of a fouled tube.

Food in its preparation has long been made subservient to the sense of taste; taste engenders appetite; and appetite in turn engenders excess. Attention is again called to the distinction to be made between appetite and hunger. Most human beings never know the sensation of true hunger, but feed their bodies at the habit-call of abnormal desire. And because of almost universal violation of the natural law of nutrition through overeating, the latter vice, apparent though it be, and distressing in its effects as it is, calls for correction as does no other in the long list of offenses against nature.

From time to time many earnest seekers have advanced beliefs and theories tending to develop a panacea for disease, but thus far without success. It is conceivable that disease may be eradicated from the world, for nature deals but in cause and effect, and the tendency in all life is towards perfect bodily balance, without which health is not. One truth, however, may here be succinctly stated: disease in all of its forms may be prevented, and in many instances, once developed, it may be cured. And the first and paramount law of its prevention is discovered in the rule that governs the quantity as well as the quality of the food supply of the human body.

In the life of man tradition, inheritance, and education combine to foster and preserve doctrines that are misleading. And in no manner is this so well illustrated as in the application of orthodox methods for the relief of bodily ills. To accept human testimony, even conscientious human testimony, as easily as men usually do is to be gullible. And this is true of the testimony of science as well as of that of the general observer. The worth of what we put into our minds or into our stomachs is of consequence to us all, and nothing can be more of a satire than the fact that, during an age when science and invention have done so much for the material world, our bodies included, the processes of the human mind, the nature of our ideas and beliefs, are so neglected that few of us ever think of our own capability of giving testimony that is true; and still fewer of us pay any attention to the daily intake of the testimony of others, which is sometimes consciously false, but which many times is more or less unconsciously inaccurate.

One reason for this lowering of mental guard is that most men possess gregarious intellects. If what is advanced seems to concur with whatever the mass mind believes, the common way is to accept it. No effort is required. Or, perhaps, there is the desire to believe—that dangerous and almost universal quality of the intellect. Because of this, one often accepts a fallacy and rejects a truth. Because of this, one reaches out for fads—mental, medical, mysterious—which give hope that the blame for weaknesses may be passed to some agency other than our own. And because of the gregarious mind and of the desire to believe, the power of mere assertion acquires its potency.

By what has been said, it must not be imagined that the incontestible learning and probity of able and reputable investigators is at all questioned. But we are privileged to doubt, and, if investigation warrants, to deny the doctrines which are generally regarded as authoritative, even though these doctrines are advanced by eminent scientists.

In the popular mind disease inculcates fear, and, when certain symptoms are in evidence, it is fled from in terror. This attitude is to be supposed so long as present general conceptions and teachings prevail, but the day is at hand when human ailments will be regarded in their true light as the means by which nature works to restore health, as the only rational processes of cure. To emphasize—disease is not a foe to life, but is the plan of nature instituted to restore a system in unbalance to equilibrium or health. That the general conception of disease and its treatment through attack upon symptoms, are wrong, and that health lies within reach of all ailing bodies that are not suffering from structural organic defect, are truths which, it is hoped, the text will fully demonstrate.

Despite prevalent belief, disease never strikes suddenly, but is the consequence of long-continued violation of natural law. It is the result of a gradual clogging of the avenues through which vitality functions, a long-drawn process of stifling the forces of life. "Every disease," says Dr. Edward Hooker Dewey, "is an inherited possibility, which every violation of the laws of life tends to develop. It is never simply an attack on a well person, but is rather a summing-up of the more or less life-long violations of health laws." Because of these transgressions, loss of digestive power occurs; lowered vitality succeeds; and disease symptoms become apparent along lines of least physical resistance.

Symptoms of disease, the tangible evidences of its presence, vary with temperament, hereditary tendencies, surroundings, and the organic state, congenital or otherwise, of the individual. No two human beings ever express in disease identical morbid signs, even under like environment; and the reason underlying the development of symptoms differing in character in persons presumably of like constitution and with the same environment is to be sought most probably in the domain of the phenomena of heredity.

Exercising the privilege of the investigator, the author

not only questions the doctrine embodied in what is known as the "germ theory" of the causation of disease, but she denies its validity. And, using in her turn the power of assertion, she condemns the remedies advanced by therapists for the cure of so-called microbically caused illnesses as being radically erroneous, leading not to health and long life, but to further disease and ultimate death.

The germ, we know, is omnipresent; it is the scavenger of animate existence; and life could not exist in its absence. In health, when physical balance is the rule, various kinds of micro-organisms live and propagate within the human body, but only to the degree necessary for the consumption of noxious products of systemic refuse, which otherwise would cause toxication. To this extent the germ is an ally of the eliminative organs, working to render harmless body waste during the time it is retained within the organism. Given for attention waste in excess of normal, germ life increases, the products of germ life add to the putrefying mass, and the task of consumption proving too great for even myriad bacilli to accomplish, physical balance is disturbed, and disease appears.

Infection is one of the methods of nature for relieving the living organism of any non-usable organic matter that may find its way into the blood, and the category of what is non-usable includes all coagulable material from serum albumen to what are known as the white corpuscles. There is doubt that virtually amounts to certainty in the mind of the author concerning the accepted theory of the life and office of the much vaunted leucocyte or white corpuscle of the blood. This body, which by scientists is given the high position of being the primordial animal cell, is in reality here placed upon the defensive, and its proponents must give proof that it is either what they claim; a vigilant policeman, a phagocyte or germ-destroyer, a tissue-builder; or that it is a surpassingly harmful foreign body that paves the way for all disease.

What we *know* about this inhabitant of the blood current is that in *good health,* when by microscopic examination we discover one thousand or thereabouts of red corpuscles in the blood, relatively we find only one or at most several white corpuscles; and, when disease appears, at first these leucocytes are unusually numerous, increasing in number with the gravity of the symptoms. If the case progresses to the point of death or its immanency, the increase of white corpuscles becomes so great as to form a complete reversal of the proportion between the red and the white which is the rule in health. And the fact is that the greater the number of these so-called phagocytes or germ-destroyers that a sick man carries in his circulation, the less probable is his chance of recovery.

If white blood corpuscles were both phagocytes and tissue builders, why do they not succeed more often in their offices, and why should they be more numerous in disease than in health, Scientists claim motion and even independent life for this whitish body in the blood; may we not suppose that its motility is due to the forces of death—to the processes of chemical disintegration?

If it be true that current teaching is open to doubt, and if, as we think it is, the criticism of the leukocyte presented is well founded, what must be the conclusion reached when we analyze the results of the past seventy-five years of study of the white blood corpuscle, It cannot be other than that nature, the greatest of all magicians, has been deceiving the elect of the scientific world by performing in their presence the feat of causing a particle of decaying organic matter to simulate life with marvelous accuracy. And, what does disease mean, if it is not that then the living organism is engaged in a life or death struggle, which has for its sole object the dislodgement, the expulsion, the annihilation of these white blood cells?

And all that is here said is in perfect consonance with the thesis of the text. For, reverting to infection, to the theory of the germ-causation of disease, it is seen that, while the process of purification that is implied by disease is essentially necessary, it is dangerous as well. While it is true that the system must be relieved of its burden of obstructing and noxious material, it is also true that the introduction of infective bacilli into a body which is carrying a large amount of waste will have substantially the same effect that a spark would have upon a heap of dry shavings in a closet—the destruction of the shavings and very probably of the house. That is to say, the fire started in the body by infective organisms, benevolent in its purpose though it be, may prove destructive to tissue and to life itself. And this, not because the organisms are themselves necessarily harmful to vitality, but because the accumulation of decomposition to be removed is so great, and the tissues in which it is located are so devitalized because of interference with their nutrition, that these structures cannot offer sufficient resistance to the destroying mob, and they therefore become involved in the disintegrating process. In other words, the body becomes the victim of the agencies actually intended for its preservation.

Before science became obsessed with the germ theory, nature conducted her own inoculating clinic, and the fight for life was then a more or less evenly balanced struggle. Since the introduction of artificial inoculation, vaccines and serums now aid in adding fuel to the flame, and in further overcoming natural resistance to disease.

We have referred many times herein to the appearance during a fast of mucus in the discharges from the body. This phenomenon is in some cases continuous throughout abstinence, although individual characteristics and conditions modify the exudation in higher or lower degree. While all of the mucosa is invariably involved in this catarrhal demonstration, the walls of the intestinal canal receive the maximum deposit, not only because of the extent of mucus membrane included in their length, but because the intestines, the colon in particular, form the main eliminative outlet of the organism.

Morgulis in his *Fasting and Undernutrition* comments on page 212 upon the very evident rapid diminution in the number of white corpuscles of the blood during the successive stages of a fast. On page 214 he says:—"The thing of particular significance with regard to the leueopenia (diminution of white corpuscles) of inanition is that while the blood is losing its white cells, the mucus membranes of the intestinal canal and the underlying tissues become infested with leucocytes. They occur either singly or in masses. According to Mingazzini, in the absence of food, leukocytes not merely accumulate in the intestinal wall but actually penetrate the mucous membrane and aggregate in the lumen *where they ultimately disintegrate.*" And he concludes that the phenomenon of this "emigration" of leucoeytes is to be viewed in the light of an increased permeability of the cell membrane to bacteria under the influence of inanition.

It is to be noted that all of the observations made by Morgulis and by those investigators whom he quotes as authorities upon inanition subjected to their experiments only animals in the normal state of function—animals and human beings in health. It is manifest that, while these observations possess interest and value in respect of the physiological and chemical changes that occur in inanition forced upon an organism that is presumably fully carrying out the transformations characteristic of normal life, their worth is doubtful when one attempts to apply the conclusions reached to the results obtained when the fast is employed as a therapeutic measure, when abstinence from food is undertaken in the presence of disease.

However, upon one point agreement may be conceded: the elimination of mucus, of pathogen, of so-called white corpuscles of the blood, is a characteristic result of abstinence from food either in health or in disease. We have stated that in disease the effort of nature is to relieve the living organism of all non-usable organic matter that finds its way into the blood, and we have here a most vivid illustration of the method which she pursues—a method in action in health to preserve the resistive qualities of the organism; in action in disease to restore the organism to the resistive condition it possesses in health.

And the result: at the completion of a scientifically conducted fast, mucus ceases to be deposited upon the walls of the intestines and other membranous surfaces, while white corpuscles have virtually disappeared from the blood stream.

Morgulis still further assists our argument by stating on page 193: "A subject still very imperfectly known, but one which merits a most careful investigation, is the *increase* in resistance to infection revealed by organisms which are recovering from inanition. Roger andJosué report such an increased tolerance towards bacilli cold in rabbits which had undergone a preliminary fast of five to seven days. The inoculation with the bacterial culture took place three to eleven days after the fast was broken. In each case the control rabbits succumbed to the infection, while all the rabbits which had previously fasted survived the inoculation. These experiments, however, need verification." This verification we shall proceed to give.

While the author was in practice in New Zealand, the world-wide epidemic of influenza of 1918 occurred. Despite its reputation for model legislation, New Zealand is not to be lauded as a mass observer of the laws of hygiene, either from the general sanitary viewpoint or from a dietetic standard. In fact, in these two respects the Dominion is remarkably lax. In consequence the influenza took mortal toll of the inhabitants of the islands, perhaps in greater proportion than occurred in any other part of the then infected world.

In corroboration of the truth contained in the substance of the paragraph just quoted from *Fasting and Undernutrition,* not one of the patients who underwent or was undergoing a fast under direction of the author, irrespective of a condition of either partial or complete recovery from disease of whatever symptomatic form, was attacked by influenza. And none among the members of the families of her clientele, past and present at the time, all of whom in their fear of infection were impelled to apply at least the less drastic elements of treatment as embodied in a light dietary, daily enemata, and cleansing baths, and all of whom were daily in contact with infected subjects, fell victim to the epidemic catarrh.

Diet 17

Perversion of Taste and Smell:

Thorough Mastication:

Should Flesh be Eaten?

Diet at any time is largely a matter of special need, but it would seem that, after a course of fasting, the successful issue of which in functional derangement embraces restoration to physiological normal, certain fixed rules might be laid down to apply to all cases. But not so. Peculiar limitations are encountered in each individual, for which individual dietetic errors coupled with physiological idiosyncrasies transmitted from generations of ancestors are responsible. Hence empirical methods must be employed in the selection of foods requisite for the case in hand.

The sense of smell, reaching out beyond the body ere food material passes the lips, assists in its selection, and this sense and taste, when normal in function and not vitiated by cultivation and habit, form a perfect picket line of protection against the introduction of unwholesome substances into the system. Normally constituted bodies prefer those odors that are classed as pleasant, yet continued contact with emanations that are distinctly disagreeable, first brings tolerance and finally pleasure in their presence. Perhaps this departure from natural law and normal instinct can be illustrated in convincing form by contemplating the sensual delight of the epicure in cheeses of doubtful age but of indubitable rottenness.

Taste also plays an important part in the choice of food material in health, and it is popularly believed that, when an article of sustenance is not repugnant to this sense, it is healthful and wholesome, and that harm cannot result from its ingestion. One of the objects that nature has in placing the nerves of taste in the mouth is that of a protective measure to prevent noxious substances from entering the stomach; but because of persistent cultivation this sense has been perverted and most men and women are more or less abnormal in taste perception. To perversion in this respect is due much of carelessness in mastication. Improperly accomplished mastication prepares a fertile soil in which the seeds of disease are promptly sown and as promptly flourish. With normal taste development the medical profession would be at a loss to administer the average drug were the patient to masticate or insalivate its substance. Recognizing this, the physician in introducing his alleged remedy into the system obviates the difficulty by the use of capsules or by injecting the drug directly into the veins.

The fallacy of attempting practical application of a

theory of food selection based upon the senses of taste and smell alone is easily demonstrable. The question resolves itself into one concerning the needs of the body, but, however, after a fast, taste and smell are restored to normal acuity and, so long as they are not abused and remain in this state, they may be used as partial indicators. At this time all wholesome food gives delight and is desired with a hunger created in a clean and healthy system that craves for nourishment and that fully enjoys its ingestion. Simple foods, properly prepared and correctly proportioned as to the relative amounts of fats, carbohydrates, and protein, with the necessary mineral salts, are what the dietitian and the subject should endeavor to supply. The fast is ended, the system is cleansed, and the digestive organs are in full vigor, waiting to form pure blood and pure tissue from pure food.

No detail further than that already disclosed is needed to show that mankind habitually overeats, and that, as a result, nutritive material is absorbed into the general circulation in quantity beyond the requirements of the body, loading the system with an unnecessary and harmful burden and hampering with poisonous waste the operation of its machinery. But, just as the liver stands guard, in so far as it may, over matter absorbed, and just as it separates good from bad, so at the very inception of the digestive process, the mouth, with its armor of teeth and its salivary apparatus, determines in large degree the amount of food needed in nutrition.

The mouth holds the nerves of taste, taste is enjoyed in the mouth, and taste has its great purpose in deciding just when food has been ground between the teeth sufficiently to prepare it for subsequent processes. Taste virtually disappears when food has been properly insalivated, and too thorough mastication cannot occur, for the benefits derived are immeasurable, even apart from the comminution of solids. The mouth easily accomplishes this work when the habit of mastication has been acquired, but, if it perform it carelessly, the other organs of digestion cannot act in normal function, and perfect digestion cannot occur, since one of its processes has been omitted. And again, the only portion of the operation of digestion that can be voluntarily controlled is that which is done in the mouth, hence the subject of the mastication of food is an all important one. Its value in the economy of the human body is excellently treated by the late Horace Fletcher in his *A-B-C of Our Own Nutrition.*

Fletcher says:

"When food is filtered into the body after having become liquefied and made alkaline or at least neutral by saliva, the appetite is given a chance to measure the needs of the body and to discriminate against excess. As soon as the point of complete saturation of any one deficiency is reached, appetite is cut off as short as possible, with no indication of stomach fullness. It will welcome a little of protein, and then turn to sugar or fat in some of their numerous forms. Thirst for water will assert itself for a moment, sometimes asking but a drop and again for a full glass; and afterwards, when near the point of complete saturation, appetite will hesitate for a moment, as if searching around for some rare substance and may find its final satisfaction in a single spoonful of sweet, or of a sip of something in sight.

"The appetite, satisfied by the infiltering process, is a sweetly appeased appetite, calm, rested, contented, normal. There is no danger from the flooding of intemperance for there is not even toleration of excess, either of more food or of more drink, and this contented appetite will remain in the condition of contentment until another need has really been earned by evaporation or destructive catabolism.

Fletcher uses in his description the term, appetite, in the sense that the word, hunger, is employed in the text. In the conditions that he so well expresses lies the solution of the problem of overeating. Mastication, carried to the degree that taste is neutralized, absolutely precludes eating save for the needs of metabolism. The supply is made equal to the demand, neither more nor less; and intemperance in food or in drink is effectively prevented. The moral attached to the excerpt quoted makes of thorough mastication a lesson to be taught in childhood, knowledge that should be transmitted from parent to offspring with more than the usual concern.

A scientific discussion of the question of diet is manifestly out of place in this text. Authorities differ widely and none has dealt with feeding from the viewpoint met after a fast, with a system, so to speak, rejuvenated. But it is no undue iteration again to point out that diet is largely a matter of special need, and that no fixed rules may be promulgated to apply in every instance. But certain general principles require discussion, of which the first and most important deals with the use or non-use of meat. Flesh in any form need never enter the dietary of normal man. Arguments for and against a meat diet have long been exchanged, and advocates of the strongest will combat the nonflesh regimen for years to come. The syllogism in refutation contains among others the following premises. First, dead animal tissue holds within it the products of metabolism. The process of change is suddenly arrested when the animal is killed, and the juices of its body contain uneliminated toxic products that no process of cooking can destroy. For that matter, even though they were completely annihilated, flesh is still changed vegetable tissue with the waste of the process of change and that of the living organism retained in its structure, a condition that logically suggests the consumption of the plant rather than of its creation. Armsby has shown that when we feed grain and other food to cattle and to sheep and then kill them for meat we recover only a very small percentage of the food values we fed them. Hence had we eaten the cattle and sheep food ourselves, instead of feeding it to the animals, we should get approximately thirty times the food value that is obtained by eating the beef and mutton supplied. In addition, decomposition of animal flesh begins at the moment of death, and by the time it is consumed as food, decay has progressed sometimes to the point of putrefaction.

Otto Carqué in his *Errors of Bio-Chemistry* says:

"There is also a marked physiological difference between plant and animal food. Animals are distinguished from vegetables by incessant decay in every tissue, a decay which is proportional to animal activity. This incessant decay necessitates incessant repair, so that the animal body has been likened to a temple on which two opposite forces are at work in every part, the one tearing down, the other repairing the breach as fast as it is made. In plants no such incessant decay has ever been discovered. If it exists at all, it must be very trifling in comparison. Protoplasm, it is true, is taken from the older parts of the plant, and these parts die; but the protoplasm does not seem to decompose, but is used again for tissue building. Thus the eternal activity of animals is of two kinds, tissue-destroying and tissue-building, while that of plants is principally of one kind, tissue-building. Flesh foods will, therefore, impart less vitality to our system than plant foods, because the former always contain a quantity of substances which have undergone the various stages of catabolism and have lost their vital force. We feel drowsy and indolent after a heavy meal of meat, while an apple, an orange, a bunch of grapes, instantly refreshes us. The theories that flesh makes flesh, that blood is converted into blood, that calf's or sheep's brain increases our mental capacity, that meat is predigested plant food, cannot stand in the light of physiological chemistry."

Experiments carried out most thoroughly by Irving Fisher, Professor of Political Economy at Yale University, show beyond any chance of refutation that the physical endurance of the human body is increased to the utmost by a non-flesh diet. In the course of these experiments meat-eating athletes competed in test exercises with non-meat eaters, both sedentary and active in occupation. The results were so largely in favor of the non-flesh dietary that the most ardent advocates of the opposite side can find no loophole through which to escape from the facts.

No adequate explanation is as yet available of the evident superiority of a vegetarian dietary over one of flesh as regards endurance, save, perhaps, in the theory that a diet composed in greater part of proteid produces uric acid and other crystalline substances, which in turn cause muscular fatigue in exercise. The facts are patent in the instances related, as well as in experiments made by the author along similar lines during the past twenty years. The results obtained have invariably demonstrated that a non-flesh dietary builds a consistently strong and enduring physical structure, while the reverse is true in great part when meat figures largely in the list of foods ingested. In the past truths such as this have been obscured because the idea contained in the term, "vegetarian," suggested what was popularly regarded as fanaticism carried beyond all bounds. This is but another exemplification of the small effect that doctrines advanced with polemical warmth coupled with enthusiasm have upon the scientific world, and for this reason the matter needs to be approached deliberately and dispassionately, and with the seriousness befitting a subject that is of more practical import than is any other in the whole range of hygienic research. When this shall have been accomplished, the theory embodied in the results of the tests mentioned will be fully borne out and conclusively established as a living truth.

With the individual himself rests the selection of a healthful and properly distributed food supply. In order to maintain a normal body in perfect equilibrium, the amount and the selection of food require careful consideration. Quantity depends upon physical characteristics and the kind of labor at which the subject is employed. A working man destroys more tissue in shorter time than does the banker or the clerk; yet, usually, the latter eat no fewer meals nor less at a sitting than does their burly brother. What is needed for the one is far more than sufficient for the others. Should the brain worker devote spare time to outdoor recreation or to manual labor a mean might be established; but, in general, equilibrium is seldom reached, and the supply of food is far in excess of requirement. The laboring man, too, is at fault in this respect, for, unless his be an exceptional case, the basis of his diet is starch, which, in addition to the unbalance produced, carries its nutritive principle in a bulky vehicle, demanding extra labor from the digestive tract in order to separate waste from nutriment and to eliminate the former.

To reduce the supply of food to the basis of demand, the plan that suggests the omission of the midday meal is perhaps the easiest to follow, and, once the habit is acquired, this repast is scarcely missed. Hunger should determine the hours for the ingestion of food each day. Regularity of habit as to the times for serving meals is an outgrowth of economic convenience, and, more often than not, the participant is imposing a burden upon a system in no need, therefore with no desire of sustenance. In health, dependent upon occupation, hunger makes demand not more than twice daily, if previous desire has been satisfied. Hunger, like the reproductive instinct, is stimulated by the changing chemistry of the body and can be satisfied only by achieving its primary purpose, the taking of food for constructive metabolism.

The late war taught us many things connected with dietetic habit. The Danes, for instance, kept healthy upon a most restricted diet. Their death rate was exceptionally low in spite of many privations. They lived on a ration that consisted very largely of vegetables and whole wheat or grain breads. And they ate very little milk and meat.

The Germans proved that it is possible to live on a diet that contains a great deal of fiber. So far as their adults were concerned, health was improved by the very low diet—at least it was not impaired. The lean German was healthier than was the pot-bellied German of pre-war days. These experiences prove that man can stand a serious cut in his food over long periods of time without permanent damage. :But the text carries out this thought in its entirety, and all that is offered from sources apart merely serves in corroboration of the truths presented.

In much that has been written concerning the matter of diet there are so many sweeping statements, so many conflicting processes of proof, impossible rules, and foolish conclusions, that no wonder is felt that the whole subject is usually ignored as too intricate. There are many who try to enforce personal ideas upon others in this connection; very persistent people these, to whom the term, "crank," may well be applied, and a "crank," who has picked up some scientific jargon and who thinks himself cured of his ailments, works more harm than good in the world. This class may be extended to include those who really have been benefited by a diet that happens to suit personal requirement, and it comprises also the one-food people who are in continual search of what not to devour, with the idea of reducing the universe to whole wheat and pecans. These people at each encounter with their fellow-men discover in the latter disease symptoms identical with their own, and insist that the remedy to which they have had recourse shall be applied. It is absurd for any who are not familiar with the chemistry of foods to endeavor to talk learnedly of their action in human physiological economy, and it may be taken as an axiom that, within the individual capability, which can be known only by individual experiment, a diet limited to not more than three proportioned items at each meal is more conducive to health than is one where unlimited choice or a single dish is the rule. A list that is limited strictly to few things trains the stomach to adapt itself accordingly, and trouble ensues when change is attempted. It is also to be remarked that when the organism has been accustomed to the digestion of animal protein, change to vegetable compounds may discover organic resistance this because of habit, for actually no essential difference exists between these two muscle building combinations excepting in origin.

After all, the amount of food and the kind of food are of secondary importance to the organic ability or inability of the individual to function. It must continually be borne in mind that in the condition of the digestive organs lies the crux of the situation. Hence the aim of both physician and patient should constantly be directed at the restoration of the system to health, after which its maintenance in this condition requires proper attention to selection and to quantity of food.

Note

Tomato Soup.

Strain one quart can of tomatoes through a coarse kitchen sieve, assisting the process by using the back of a heavy spoon. This serves to separate seeds and skin from juice and pulp. Add to the latter a dessert-spoon of butter or corn oil, and heat but do not boil. If desired, a small quantity of honey may be used. F'or breaking a fast this broth is excellent food, and one coffee-cup taken four times at regular intervals should suffice for the first day succeeding abstinence. The quantity taken may be increased on the second day to one pint eaten morning and evening with other food material gradually added as previously described.

If ripe tomatoes from the garden are used instead of the canned variety, simmer the fruit until tender, but at no point in cooking allow to boil, since high temperature tends to destroy the vitamins with which this fruit is so richly furnished. After cooking, strain and gauge proportions as with the canned fruit.

Rest and Recuperation 18

Muscular Rest:

Best for the Digestive Organs:

The Hibernating Animals:

The Hunger Strke of Mcswiney and Others

Muscular tissue is continually undergoing change in structure. The cells that form it are constantly dying, are cast off, and fresh material for their rebuilding is being supplied. The waste resulting, if retained, is systemically harmful; and, in order to permit of its elimination and replacement with wholesome cell pabulum, muscular rest must occur. Not only does this apply to muscles in super-active use, but to those of all of the bodily fabric. Rapid exercise of any part of the human machine can be continued but for a short time, for, because of vigorous muscular action, voluntary or involuntary, cells are rapidly broken down, their poisonous waste is thrown into the blood, and is carried to the remotest portions of the organism. Every organ of the body is thus deleteriously affected, and resulting symptoms of self-toxication appear that may end disastrously. The only means of recuperation lies in muscular rest.

The heart, although making contractions at the rate of seventy-two beats a minute, is able to continue its work throughout the life of the individual, since each contraction of this muscle is followed by a slight interval of rest, during which its cells recuperate. Stimulate the heart beat beyond its normal rate, and a point is soon reached at which poisonous products from broken-down cells are not carried away with sufficient rapidity, while regeneration is defectively performed, since the intervals of rest are inadequate. Similar conditions are met when the muscles used in respiration, those of the chest, the diaphragm, and the abdomen, are overworked.

The muscles that move involuntarily, those that are not subject to the human will, never know absolute rest, for they continue their labors whether the body be asleep or awake. On the other hand, those muscles, the action of which depends upon brain direction, cannot work continuously, lest fatigue with fatal exhaustion follow. Seemingly, automatic labor, labor not directed by volition, does not wear. It is only conscious work that requires for recuperation and muscle rebuilding non-use or physical rest. This is permitted in that loss of consciousness regularly recurrent in animal life, which is called sleep.

Physical growth and muscular development in man

are never completely rounded out, and this may be attributed to a double cause. Theoretically, every muscle of the body should be exercised impartially and should be nourished with the exact amount of cell pabulum that is needful for the replacement of its broken-down substance. These conditions are virtually never fulfilled. That they may be is a possibility to be contemplated with surety, since they are logical conclusions based on natural law. To bring them to consummation, reciprocal active relation must exist between intake and outgo, rebuilding and waste, labor and rest, consciousness and sleep.

The processes of nutrition are involuntary in character so long as material suitable for their accomplishment is furnished for their use, but they may be directed in part by the individual to the extent of the preparation and of the selection in kind and quantity of food required. When the function of digestion becomes impaired, disease results. And functional disease is analogous to muscular fatigue; hence, since nature includes in her law of recuperation both systemic purification and organic rest, it is reasonable to assume what the text promulgates: organic rest through abeyance of the processes of digestion and assimilation, with consequent systemic cleansing and renewal of normal functional activity.

The manner in which the digestive organs and those allied to them may be given needed rest is to the mass mind perhaps not at once apparent. The mere thought of abstention from food carries with it repudiation of the long-taught doctrine that frequent feeding both in health and in illness is needful for the maintenance of vitality and strength. Yet just this omission of food is meant when rest for overworked organs is suggested. The phenomena of fasting for the cure of disease include facts that prove that the human body does not depend for strength or for vitality solely upon food ingested; the latter is in the main utilized for the repair of the fabric of the body; by means of food the material framework is kept in condition to permit of the liberation of energy in its variety of manifestation. The body, then, is but a vehicle for the expression of the life principle. But the life principle itself is an entity, operating through its vehicle only so long as its lines of transmission are unobstructed by the causes of disease.

Diminution in weight, often excessive, always occurs in illness, even though food is ingested. (Exceptions with obese or dropsical symptoms noted.) In itself this shows that nature is proceeding with her process of purification, despite the obstacles in her path, and that she is protecting the body by inhibiting the function of assimilation. This she will continue to do until the avenues for the passage of vital force are partially or wholly cleared, or until organic defect beyond repair is uncovered. In the former event, health will eventually be restored; in the latter, the death of the body is presaged.

Also, when disease is present, under the more prevalent methods, feeding is continuous in accordance with the doctrine that nourishment is at all times necessary to "keep up strength." If the stomach rebel, other organs are assailed with the idea of conveying through them the nutriment considered necessary, and this in spite of very evident protests on the part of bodily function. The question naturally suggests itself: why, if food is constantly supplied, does the body lose in weight! This query was covered in a previous chapter, but its answer is found in the fact that in disease intake of food is not properly digested, is consequently incapable of complete and healthful assimilation, and, far from acting as constructive material for tissue regeneration, proves an added systemic burden and a source of toxication. Another cause of loss of weight, slighter in degree, is discovered in that brain and nerve tissue, as instruments for the expression of thought, motion, and sensation, are protected from deterioration in substance by that provision of nature which permits them to utilize nourishment stored in the interstices of tissue. This they consume in illness and in health, and, when in disease normal balance is disturbed, when body tissue is not rebuilt as is the case in health, nerve substance is still supported from the same source of supply.

With slight differences the physiology of digestion in all mammals is markedly similar. In disease the lower mammalia abstain from food until hunger returns, when health is rapidly recovered. To this they are impelled by instinct, by animal sagacity, a faculty implanted by nature in the whole of animate creation. The fasts which animals instinctively undergo in disease are phenomena which cannot help but be constantly observed, but which are not in general intelligently perceived. A common expression in reference to illness in the horse embodies the phrase, "off his feed," and this negation on the part of the animal confirms the existence an instinctive sense that impels it to fast when its physical well-being is overturned. And this natural spontaneous impulse is not confined to mammals, for birds, reptiles, in fact the whole animal kingdom, abstain from food when ailing. A python in captivity has been known to fast for thirteen months, with great loss in weight, it is true, but with eventual recuperation and recovery. And cats and canines often prolong abstention to skeleton condition, after which strength and vitality progressively increase until normal is again attained. Instances such as these may be multiplied indefinitely.

While not occasioned by the invasion of disease, it is interesting to note in this connection that condition of lethargy undergone by certain animals during the winter months, known as hibernation, a condition in which the functions of the body are in great measure suspended. How a warm-blooded animal used to the most stirring activities during eight or nine months of the year can retire to a den, and from an ordinary sleep, which it is at first, pass into a condition of torpor in which all the organs that have to do with digestion, assimilation, and waste, excepting the lungs, suspend their functions and remain quiescent for a period of several months, is more or less a sealed book to science.

In man and the non-hibernating animals the action of the body functions are continuous awake or asleep, but in the bear, the marmot, the prairie dog, during the hibernating period, the functions of digestion, assimilation, and elimination are suspended until the animal awakens in the spring.

A bear, if sufficiently fat, begins to fast some weeks before he retires to winter quarters; but, if there has been lack of food, or, if the animal is old, with poor teeth, it will eat to the very day of entering its den, and this last meal will be found in the stomach when the revival from winter sleep takes place.

The average bear at the beginning of hibernation is covered with a layer of fat that varies from two to six inches in thickness, and, if the animal is killed at this time and the fat removed from the carcass, the latter is found plump and full-fleshed. But, killed after some months in the den, a heavier layer of fat is discovered, with a diminution in lean flesh, which by this time has become lax and flabby in texture. The carcass, then stripped of its fat, will be noticeably smaller than that of a bear of similar size killed in the fall or in the early winter.

There is then evidently a continual process of change from nitrogenous to carbonaceous tissue proceeding while the winter sleep of the hibernating animal endures; and, in this transmutation of muscle into fat, lies perhaps the secret of the torpor in which the bear is wrapped.

For, when a bear first goes into his den, his sleep is natural, and he is easily aroused. But, left undisturbed, sleep develops into stupor; respiration and circulation are the only evidences of life, and they are both retarded in action. Carbon resulting from the change of protein into fat within the system, is retained in the blood, because all of the organs of elimination, excepting the lungs, are without function; and respiration is so slow that there is continuously an excess of carbonic acid gas in the blood stream, and a consequent condition of toxication, of torpor.

At times during hibernation the female bear will bring her young into the world, and then milk is elaborated in amount sufficient to maintain the cubs. The birth of young and the physiological chemistry of continued milk production in the fasting, torpor-ridden bear have particular interest here, analogous as these phenomena are to the related cases in the text of pregnant women proceeding to confinement, but fasting for weeks the while.

A hibernating bear never soils his den with urine or ordure, for no waste is formed, consequently none is voided. But, after the period of winter sleep is over, the animal feeds ravenously upon young clover and grass, and extreme purging results, with succeeding rapid reduction of the fatty tissue formed as described while coma lasted.

A certain degree of cold is necessary before a bear can hibernate, but, in so far as may be ascertained, body temperature remains at standard during the experience. That is, the animal is warm to the touch, although it is in a state of constant shivering. Analogy is again evident between this condition and what is termed herein "fasters' chilliness."

Omitting from consideration mental conditions, such as fear and worry, which of necessity react upon the physical body, and setting aside severe and more or less continuous physical suffering, the average human being cannot die from lack of food for several months. This statement of fact is verified constantly in the employment of fasting as a therapeutic measure, and it has recently been brought to public attention and conclusively substantiated in instances to which reference is now made.

It would appear that the medical profession in whole or in greater part has been egregiously in ignorance of the resources of the human body when for any cause it is denied nourishment. The various encyclopedias, notably *Britannica,* until revisions were made in 1921, carried articles on inanition and fasting, which asserted over medical signature that from ten to fourteen days marked the extreme limit to which the human body would endure in the absence of food. In other words, starvation and death would occur were nourishment denied for approximately the period of time named. While doubt may have existed in the minds of the more advanced among the medical fraternity, revision of these articles was definitely occasioned only by the comparatively recent "hunger strike" of Terence McSwiney, former Lord Mayor of Cork, Ireland, and of several of his political colleagues.

The charge upon which Lord Mayor McSwiney was convicted, and for which he was sentenced to two years in Brixton prison, England, was that of sedition against British government. He began to serve his sentence in August, 1920, and upon his incarceration, in protest against what he considered an unjust trial and conviction, he refused to eat. In spite of constant persuasion and attempts at forced feeding, McSwiney's fasting continued until October 25th, 1920, a period of seventy-four days, when his death occurred. McSwiney was quite cognizant of the details of the method of fasting for the cure of disease, and in so far as was possible in prison surroundings, he made use of the hygienic accessories that are described herein. His familiarity with the writings of the author of this text accounted for the knowledge that permitted him to continue his fast without succumbing for two and one-half months. McSwiney might, and, in the opinion of the writer, would have lived longer had it not been that, in the latter days of his life, he became too weak to prevent efforts on the part of the jail physician to force food upon him, and, when he lapsed into unconsciousness because of strength overstrained and nerves tensed beyond limit through resistance, strychnine was injected into his veins as a heart stimulant, and he died.

Of McSwiney's political colleagues, also imprisoned and also on "hunger strike," one died after sixty-eight days of fasting, while the others all endured until McSwiney's death and after. It is reported that one of these men continued his fast for the extremely lengthy period of ninety days. And it is to be noted that, with the exception of that seditionist who succumbed at the end of sixty-eight days, all of the others, who fasted much longer than McSwiney himself, resumed feeding and rapidly recuperated to a condition of body ultimately superior to that which was theirs before they undertook their "hunger strike."

Earlier in the text cases were cited that underwent abstinence from food for periods ranging from eleven to seventy-five days. And it is to be remembered that these cases resorted to the method because they were ill, and that some of them were in an extreme state of emaciation to begin with. Yet, although no food was ingested, life was supported, functional processes were restored, and recovery resulted.

In one instance, a patient of the writer during a period of 140 days fasted absolutely 118 days. This case was bedridden, and had been so for years; the body was emaciated, and chronic functional disease and confinement to bed had caused progressive wasting of the muscles. Yet, as a consequence of the bodily purification resulting from abstinence from food, not only was great relief experienced, but recovery, save in minor degree, the aftermath of muscular non-use, occurred.

If, then, the body can exist without food for an extended time, and, if in illness the stomach instinctively objects, as it does, to ingestion, it is reasonable to infer that food not desired is not at this time necessary for bodily maintenance; and, once accepted as true, this inference is abundantly justified. The results of a practical and scientific application of the method of systemic purification defined herein are such as to lead to the conclusion that, in the absence of serious structural defects in vital organs, abstinence from food, accompanied by its natural health-restoring and health-preserving accessories, is the unfailing remedy for relief from functional ills.

Mental and Physical Action and Reaction 19

Mind Influences Function and Function Influences Mind:

A Case of Insanity:

Sick Geniuses:

The Subconscious Mind:

Muscular action in the body may be brought about in two ways—through the brain itself, or through internal or external physical causes. In both instances the nerve centers perform their functions, either in the inception of the thought or in the transfer of inward or outward cause. The act of moving the hand, for example, may originate in the brain, or it may occur because the member is in proximity to fire. In the former contingency the act begins with the thought in the brain, and nervous influence operates directly upon the muscles. In the second condition the sensory nerves inform the brain that the flesh is burning, and the brain sets in motion the muscles necessary to move the hand. In both cases the motive power emanates from the brain, and the phenomenon as observed may happen in connection with any specific portion of the body. Not only are these phenomena true of the muscles controlled by the will, but they may also be observed in similar phase in organs beyond the power of volition in function, as the heart, the lungs, and the stomach. Swallowing an emetic causes vomiting, an effect occasioned by muscular contraction of the stomach for the purpose of ejecting a substance irritating to the nerves of that organ. The mere sight or thought of a disgusting object may have the same consequence, and imagination is frequently able to produce results like those that are caused by the administration of a powerful drug or by a combination of physical conditions.

Every organic act, normal or abnormal, is due solely to a current sent from one of the great nerve centers, and the latter may be called into operation either directly by feeling or thought, or indirectly by reflex action. The mind and the emotions exercise large influence upon physical function, but the field over which that influence extends is comparatively little known. It is, in some respects, almost unbounded, for every bodily function may be hastened, retarded, or even totally suspended by the subjective effect of thought. Pleasurable emotions are physically wholesome; painful ones, the reverse; but, when too intense and sudden, either can terminate life.

The fibers of the pneumogastric nerve are distributed principally in and about the lungs and the stomach; hence its name. Whatever may be the motor functions that this nerve supplies, it has great power over the process of digestion, for, when its fibers are severed below those branches that extend to the trachea, digestion is virtually arrested. Nervous influence is essential to the proper action of the stomach, and, in the region of this organ, the nerves are so interlaced one with another that, even though the direct road be destroyed, by-paths will still remain for the passage of nerve energy. If the latter force were not needed in digestion, no reason would exist for the suspension of function by its withdrawal. This is well illustrated when it is observed that the invariable effect of worry, anxiety, fright, anger, and the like, is to arrest for a time all digestive action. Cause is obvious when the close connection that exists between the brain and the pneumogastric nerve is considered. Also, if nervous force is diverted in directions other than those pursued in the digestion of food, or if it is impeded by impingement of nerve substance at emergence from the spinal column, similar results ensue as when the pneumogastric nerve is severed.

Does the physical condition of the body in reflex affect the minds. Observation shows that it has such influence upon brain function that perfect reflection of physical condition is continuously displayed in the working of the intellect. A healthy and balanced mind can emanate only from a healthy body. The reverse is equally true.

In health the constructive and destructive changes

that take place in the human body progress without noticeable diminution or increase in excellence of brain function so long as balance between assimilation and elimination is the rule. In conditions of debility from whatever cause, but especially when the intake of food is in excess of demand, and waste is accumulated in quantity too great for disposal by the eliminative organs, absorption of poisons generated in fermenting refuse retained in the intestinal tract is continuous, and the subject becomes a victim of autointoxication, is drunk with the products of his own decomposition. This condition, long continued, is no less baneful in effect than is that of alcoholic saturation, and in some instances it takes the form of insanity, while in all diminished brain power is in evidence.

The digestion of a meal with the subsequent forcing of food waste through the bowels consumes nerve energy in amount greater than is ordinarily conceived. Some investigators go so far as to say that the process involved requires nervous expenditure in excess of that demanded in the exercise of the voluntarily controlled muscles. In any event overfeeding never fails to result in weakened vitality. In the normal subject, sufficient food, perfectly digested and assimilated, produces a body with brain power equal to clear thought, an organism with a maximum of both physical and mental energy. Food in amount more than the individual requires entails excessive labor upon the organs of digestion, drain upon nerve power, and consequent of vitality.

Barring destructive changes in brain or nerve tissue

from injury, the cause of mental disease is one and the same with that of physical unbalance. Physical signs invariably preceding mental danger signals should be heeded and remedied when first displayed. One of the simplest of these warnings is the drowsiness that overcomes the overfed. Here the nerves evince fatigue, and incidentally fatigue, both muscular and mental, is one of the safety valves of the human machine. If at this time stimulating effort is resorted to, results are always detrimental, for, as in exercise, to stifle a feeling of fatigue in order to be able to continue muscular exertion is like forcibly closing the safety gauge so that the boiler may be overheated. In other words, taking a stimulant when tired in order to whip up flagging physical or mental vigor subsequently leaves both body and mind in condition more exhausted than when the sensation of fatiguc first signaled its warning. Likewise food, which in itself is stimulating in effect, taken when either physical or mental weariness is felt, carries its own quota of detrimental consequences.

We cannot escape the conclusion that mind influences function just as function influences mind. It is also virtually axiomatic that continued functional derangement finally ends in organic disease, and organic disease gives rise to characteristic mental states that vary from the fearful anxiety of the sufferer from neuralgia of the heart to the hopeful attitude of the dying consumptive.

It is an established feet that drugs, however powerful, do not affect the structure of brain tissue; and it is equally well known that in most instances of insanity there is no apparent deterioration in quality or structure of nerve substance. In these phenomena lies strong collateral proof that the sources of mental disease are to be sought elsewhere than in the brain. Injuries and ailments that involve structural change in brain matter will necessarily interfere with brain function, and in softening of the brain and in certain forms of paralysis there are organic alterations that may be noted on dissection. But in hysteria, epilepsy, or any of the manias, no changes in structure of either brain or nerve substance can be discovered, notwithstanding the presence of extreme mental alienation.

To illustrate the effect of abnormal physical condition upon mind function, the following case is cited. The patient, a man thirty years of age, presented a history of continuous digestive trouble accompanied by melancholia. Examination pointed to the conviction that the morbid mental symptom was the result of functional inactivity of the digestive tract, complicated with decided indications of organic disease. A tentative dietary of fruits and vegetable broths afforded the relief usual when organic labor is thus lightened. But skill in observing and determining the sequelae of dietetic changes caused delay in prognosis, for it is always needful to distinguish between mitigation of the distress of disease that is temporary in character, and that which evinces progress towards recovery. Hence, though symptoms in some respects were favorable, no predication was made as to the ultimate outcome. At the end of three weeks of the regimen imposed, the major signals all pointed to organic disability of extreme gravity, and at his request for definite opinion for or against recovery, the patient was informed that there seemed no possible hope of restoration to health. He then ceased his office visits, and a month later was discovered dead by suicide, an act committed, as the condition of the body showed, within a few days after discontinuing treatment. The previous conduct of the man, his brooding depression, and the contents of a number of scribbled letters found among his effects, now definitely fixed the case as one of insanity, whatever the state of his body might prove to be. The latter was in condition such that an autopsy could be performed, and it revealed the following: the kidneys were normal; the lungs and the heart were congested, but functionally equal to their tasks; the liver was hardened, and there was but a rudimentary gall sac, which contained no bilious fluid and gave no indication that the liver had been functioning, no characteristic stain being present, the color of the sac being a chalky white; the stomach was dilated and filled with food, and glandular activity in the organ must have been inoperative for some time previous to death; the small intestines showed bleached portions that had undoubtedly been without function for an indefinite period; the transverse section of the colon was much dilated, contained a large amount of hardened feces and had fallen shaping the whole organ into a letter "M", with the vertex of the dropped portion resting upon the pelvis; it, as well as the ascending and descending parts, were adherent at their angles for several inches; the bladder was apparently normal; the pancreas was a soft degenerated mass; the spleen was hardened; the mesentery exhibited old lesions, while no trace of the omentum was found; but the brain was structurally perfect.

The instance cited shows a body exceedingly deformed internally in which, despite its faulty structure, the processes of growth and maintenance progressed for thirty years. The cause of the organic defects discovered is to be attributed to digestive activity partially inhibited in early life through disease, the effects of which were very probably augmented by the use of drugs. In this case progressive inability to function produced morbid mental disturbance. It may be asked why a similar result was not observed in each of the instances related elsewhere in the text, or for that matter in any diseased human body; and reply is made that physical unbalance in any degree invariably affects mind-function, and this usually in adverse manner. But here again we enter the domain of the idiosyncrasy of individuality, of the limitations and requirements of a subject segregated from other individuals by his own constitutional peculiarities and tendencies, be these mental or physical. For instance, it is well known that there are certain temperaments that develop delirium in fever, even when the latter is mild in type, while there are others who may experience rise in body heat of as much as four or five degrees above register without sign of loss in mental equilibrium. But the close observer notes that the latter in the circumstances will exhibit certain other vagaries of the mind that are not apparent when function is normal in character.

Yet we must not neglect to mark and to ponder the other side of the question, for, as has been said, as mind influences function, so function influences mind. As an example, it is admitted that arterial strain, an undue pressure upon the walls of the arteries commonly known as high blood pressure, tends to produce a fatty degeneration of their inner coat, and thus gives rise to arterial tumors and to cerebral hemorrhage, which sometimes causes paralysis, apoplexy, and softening of the brain. Now it is certain that such tension may result from continued anxiety, and that it is the cause of many cases of angina pectoris or neuralgia of the heart, effecting those cardiac changes to which some of the forms of angina are due.

It is also well established that mental disturbance gives rise to dyspepsia, and observation and experiment show that anger and other emotions arrest the secretion of gastric juice, and that probably the peristaltic action of both stomach and intestines is likewise affected. In this connection the extreme constipation of melancholia is to be noted. Simple jaundice is often the result of sudden emotion, and it is sometimes followed by acute yellow atrophy, a wasting of the liver with yellow pigmentation. In the latter form of jaundice there is always disorganization of the cells of the liver.

A man who works with his brain after a sleepless night or when he is in the clutches of some discomforting indisposition at times does not see how he can possibly accomplish his day's stint. He attempts it, however, and is often surprised to find that he works more rapidly and with more acuity than when in normal state. This occurs because, feeling the necessity, he brings his will into play and concentrates with greater determination than usual upon what is before him. So our attention is often called to the fact, and it is a fact, that a very large percentage of the world's best work has been done by men who were not in health most of the time that they were about it. But does this offer an argument in favor of the possession of a defective unhealthy body? These very men, though we hail them as geniuses, were and are universally under the control of an impressible and capricious nervous temperament, always a handicap upon thorough and efficient accomplishment. And it is interesting to speculate upon the kind and the amount of labor with which the genius in ill health might have enriched the world had he been the possessor of a physically normal body. Would this work have been of a quality surpassing that which was produced by forced concentration; or would the physical ease of health have removed the spur of accomplishment?

We cannot, if we would not eventually fall short of our desired achievements, afford to discriminate in favor of either mind or body. The development of each is equally essential to the greatest and best results from the other. Hence, given a body free from any organic trouble, the successful enjoyment and prolongation of life is as much dependent upon intellectual development as upon physical, and vice versa.

It is thus apparent that the work that the brain can perform is in highest degree proportional to and dependent upon the physical condition of its body. To repeat, a functionally perfect brain is the product only of a physically perfect body. And it is to be emphasized that the brain is not a producer of energy, nor of vitality, nor of the mental processes. It acts but as a medium of reception and transmission, and it in itself no more thinks than do the words that express a thought. Mind, as received from the creative source, is perfect; its expression is affected by the functional ability or inability of its human instrument.

The mysterious forces, energy and vitality, which are seen manifested in the life of the body, exist outside of and independent of the human vehicle. A healthy organism is one that is in position to liberate these principles in the form of power, mental and physical, as it is needed in the activities.

Human beings possess what are known as the conscious and subconscious minds. The conscious mind controls those acts which are subject to the will and those thoughts which are produced by brain effort in conscious moments. The subconscious mind covers that which occurs without conscious perception. The conscious mind could not possibly send messages to the numerous glands that fit the body for action, nor attend to all the delicate adjustments that enter into the process. The conscious mind in most of us does not even know of the existence of the organs and secretions involved. But there is a something in mentality that is without conscious perception, and that takes advantage of all of the past, gauging means to an end with perfect nicety.

All processes of healing are subconscious. Even pain and the distressing symptoms of sickness are to be regarded as benevolent warnings that sharply remind us of our condition, and that compel the repose which we require, or that deter us from admitting into the system substances which are injurious. They not only point to the existence of a mind that is subconscious, but they indicate how great a part that mind plays in the curing of every form of disease. Anything that weakens or depresses the subconscious mind exposes us to disease by making us less able to resist its encroachments. And, on the other hand, we possess such allies and resources within ourselves that the chief function of the physician should be to awaken in his patients the will to live, and to employ every element of resistance which the system itself affords.

If humanity since its creation had constantly been caring for its individual bodies, no condition of disease could make its appearance suddenly. There could be no physical collapse, for cancers, tumors, Bright's disease, diabetes, etc., all require time to develop, and in a body that is both mentally and physically conscious, their beginnings cannot help but be observed, understood, and remedied. For he who is in the habit of caring properly for his body, who understands and obeys natural physical law, cannot for one day neglect his course of action, because, subconsciously if not consciously, he is subjected to irritation and discomfort. To illustrate, he who is used to pure air cannot endure a vitiated atmosphere, and he who bathes his body daily, in case of omission, finds his skin figuratively talking to him because of its neglect.

A diseased body is the product of a process development that began with its birth, for every symptom in its finality is cumulative. The colds and fevers of infancy and adolescence, the causes of which are imperfectly eliminated, leave their residue to accumulate until the eventual crisis occurs. And, as in the physical so in the mental realm, disease of the mind, and in it we include crime as well as insanity, are symptoms of unbalance, often produced because of physical reaction. Crime begins in small acts, develops like a cancer, and in reality it is to be regarded as a cancer of the conscious mind, and hence should be treated as is disease. Instead, society punishes the discovered victim. Insanity is but another form of unbalance that in many instances arises from functional physical disturbance, yet it, too, is handled as is crime, its sufferers being subjected to police authority in ways that are reminders of the dark ages.

And since brain troubles in great part arise from functional physical derangement, their alleviation and cure is to be sought in systemic bodily purification. The text fully covers the manner in which the latter process may best be accomplished, in fact the only way in which it can be done. And, could the fast and its hygienic accessories be introduced and scientifically administered in all asylums, insane as well as criminal, of the land, numbers of their inmates would be restored both in mind and in body. And further, in those in whom mental incapacity is due to organic structural defects that hamper normal function, the form and degree of the latter would at once be revealed, and the knowledge thus gained would determine to what extent treatment should be carried. And it is probable that among even these severely afflicted sufferers there might be many who could be brought to mental responsibility. Apart from its therapeutic worth, a trial of the method in public institutions offers two other points of merit, viz., it would ameliorate much of the suffering now undergone by stimulated unruly patients who need restraint, and it would lower by many thousands of dollars the expense of caring for these wards of the state. But, if not for the sake of those who pay taxes, at least for the salvation of those detained in asylums for the insane and criminal, the method is entitled to a thorough investigation and trial at the hands of government.

To many minds the thought that human life is in any way connected with or dependent upon ordinary natural agencies carries with it denial of faith in the divine. Reasoning thus, these intellects segregate in toto spirituality from materiality, refusing to recognize their manifest interdependence. A calm retrospect of the history of the Christ causes one to know that Jesus, apart from his spiritual endowment, was a man in the flesh and of the flesh; that he was subject to the laws of the body, to its necessities and to its temptations. It is written, "Jesus was led up of the spirit into the wilderness to be tempted of the devil. And when he had fasted forty days and forty nights, he was afterward an hungered."

The application of this fragment of sacred history to the subject matter of the text may not be obvious, but brief explanation will serve to show that the related incident is distinctly pertinent. Fasting the body for the sake of health was understood and followed by the older civilizations; and fasting for the attainment of that higher mentality which borders upon spirituality is still employed by the members of that system of philosophy known as Yoga, in which meditation upon the supreme spirit is inculcated as the way to final beatitude. That the Christ acquainted with and was learned in these practices is fully substantiated by the evident purpose and scientific completion of a period of forty days and nights of abstinence from food. Jesus never overturned natural law; he worked with it always, and his statement concerning prayer and fasting in disease is easy of analysis. "More things are wrought by prayer than this world dreams of." And fasting, physical in application, conduces to the highest degree of mental clarity. The body, purified of its dross, approaches more nearly the spiritual vehicle it is intended to be. Successfully conducted to the point of the return of hunger, the body and its brain are enhanced in substance and in function. In this condition difficulties are solved, decisions are made, and conclusions are reached with marvelous clearness and dispatch.

The Gospel relates that Jesus was led up into the wilderness for the purpose of being tempted—a test through which mere man passes daily, and ofttimes daily fails to meet. But Jesus, before temptation assailed, fasted for the approximate time needful for physiological purification of the adult body, and the fast concluded, we are specifically told, with its physiologically correct symptom, the return of hunger. We do not err, we think, in attributing to the Christ in the flesh the experiences of the flesh. Why else should he have been subjected to temptation? And physically there must have been need for regeneration, for the incident occurred just before the beginning of his active ministry, when all of his power of endurance was to be called forth, and mental acuity more than normal was to be commanded at every future moment of his physical life. And in addition the divine plan embodied further proof of its all-embracing wisdom in that it held up to the world divinity clothed in a material body, endowed with physical attributes, and subjected to the test of physical desire—a test that could perfectly be withstood only by a mind functioning in a body physiologically pure.

The Christ invariably worked through the material, the physical, to the mental and spiritual. And perfect spirituality in man requires its vehicle, the material body, to be physically excellent. Purity of body, purity of mind, purity of heart—these alone may commune with the divine.

Death in the Fast

20

A Theory of Death:

Eleven Cases of Death in the Fast:

Summary of Post Mortem Findings

No Fully satisfactory definition in explanation of what is called death in the physical body has ever been given. In conformity with the theory of life, upon which the belief of the author is based, a definition of physical death is offered that, following the tenets of that belief, discovers completely for her the phenomenon of the dissolution of the animal body. The theory referred to considers energy, vitality, or life force, as an entity that emanates from a source without the animal organism, and that animates the latter when, with the body as a laboratory, the chemical transformations necessary to life are effected. This means that the expression of energy as exhibited in sentient living organisms is achieved with those organisms functioning merely as means of transmission, as vehicles. While the explanation may be a bit labored, its purport should be clear, and the definition of physical death here offered is this:—when, for one reason or another, the mysterious force which permeates every sentient living body, giving to it motion, sensation, and thought, is prevented entrance to or passage through the organism, what is called death occurs. This definition is not strikingly original, nor is it completely satisfying, but, after all, the sciences have not as yet been able to analyze life nor the sources of life; and the phenomenon of its cessation, or what is called death, is just as much a mystery.

A digression may here be pardoned. Just what is to be after death, apart from what faith may predicate, we do not know. And men should fear only what they know. They should not, like children, be afraid to go to bed in the dark, afraid of things that they imagine. In all that we really know there is nothing about death to frighten us. We know that our bodies go back to the earth. We know that birth and death come alike to all of us. We can remember nothing that occurred before we were born, yet this thought is not fearsome. We know that this universe, in which the earth is but a grain of sand, is managed with marvelous wisdom and justice. We know in consequence that we have no reason to fear injustice, or terror, or torture.

Death in the physical body is to be regarded as having taken place when there is complete stoppage of the functions of the brain and of the organs of respiration and circulation, with sequent cessation of the processes dependent upon these functions. To amplify, death occurs whenever, through disease or shock, the brain, the storage battery of physical and mental life, becomes unable to perform its task of transmitting energy—

life force to its points of action or expression, the vital organs of the body. Vital organs cease functioning when there is obstruction or demolition of some portion of the main lines of transmission followed by life force in its passage from the brain. That this may happen by reason of long continued denial of food to the organism is undoubtedly true, but death from the exhaustion of inanition caused by absence of food is most rare in occurrence. On the other hand, in bodies that are continuously supplied with sustenance, exhaustion from lack of nourishment because of disorder of the nutritive functions proves a most usual agent of dissolution. And this is true since this sort of exhaustion, while having its source in the functional disability of the organs of nutrition, eventually succeeds in inhibiting the cells of the brain from acquiring and hence assimilating those substances necessary for their conservation.

In average conditions death results from disease that is functional in character, not organic. In the experience of the author, death during a fast never has occurred when merely functional disorder was present, nor did it ever result for the sole reason that food was withheld. In every instance listed in this chapter, in every instance of death that has happened during the long years of practice upon which this text is based, the cause of dissolution was conclusively shown by post mortem examination to have been the inevitable consequence of obstruction through structural defect of some portion of the avenues through which life force is expressed. And it is questionable whether, in a conscious being not afflicted with morbid impairment of tissue, or not so situated that food could not be supplied when hunger made its demand, death has resulted from starvation, or, in other words, from the exhaustion of brain sustenance. No evidence that is conclusive shows that this has ever happened.

In disease that is functional in origin and character the fast may be carried to its logical end without a particle of anxiety, for the law of hunger marks the limit beyond which abstinence may not continue lest starvation ensue. Hence, death from starvation is impossible during a fast when functional disease is in question. In the presence of structural organic deficiency the result is not assured. When, however, impairment of tissue is slight in degree, recovery is possible; but, when the fault is such that structural restoration of the organ or organs affected is beyond the power of natural law, no hope of cure exists, although, because functional labor is lessened through abstinence, and distress is with certainty relieved, life may be prolonged. It is always to be remembered that in all disease, whatever its form, the fast is nature's sole curative agency, and is then as much a function as is feeding in health.

The autopsies held upon the bodies of the subjects of whom the causes of death are here described disclosed in every instance disease that was organic in character. In most of these cases arrested development of one or more of the functioning parts of the body was discovered, and in all of them malformation of the intestines was displayed that must be attributed to long continued irritation with inflammation. These cases are those of persons who had resorted to orthodox methods for the relief of their suffering until orthodoxy proved without avail, and who only then bethought themselves of natural law.

In view of the defects exhibited, it is certain that malnutrition occurring in the developing period of life, coupled perhaps with the baneful effects of drugs administered in the attempt to remedy disease, was responsible for fatal issue. Nature had endowed each of these subjects at birth with presumably normal vitality; each of them had suffered early in life from severe forms of functional disorder; and each, with one exception, had virtually exhausted the list of medicines designated as remedies for the symptoms displayed.

While it is not at all a just concept to attempt to place entire responsibility for the conditions shown upon drug dosage, it is to be recognized that, broadly speaking, there is no drug that is in effect not a poison. It is also to be recognized that, while harm ensues when drugs are used for the suppression of disease in mature years, the consequences of administering medical remedies in infancy and in adolescence are much more detrimental.

The instances of death now to be cited occurred while a fast was in progress, or while the patient was undergoing a period of dieting. Each casts light upon the ease of diagnosis consequent upon abstinence from food as a therapeutic measure; while the autopsies also disclose the deleterious effects upon the human body of dietetic errors and of drug treatment. In every case the cause of death is conclusively shown to have been due to the presence of structural organic defeat that was beyond repair. Two of the deaths described happened when the subjects were on a dietary, but the conditions discovered in these showed no decided differences in causation from those displayed when dissolution took place while a fast was in progress. In all of the related cases death was certain, fasting or feeding. The list is selected from a total of twenty-two fatalities occurring in a practice confined to therapeutic fasting and its accessories that covers a period of over thirty years. The number of cases handled is about thirty thousand, and each of these fasted at some time while under guidance for intervals varying from one day to seventy-five.

Case 1. A married woman, thirty-eight years of age, who had devoted twenty years in vain attempt to regain lost health under medical guidance. She finally discovered that alternating periods of dieting and abstinence from food, usually short in duration, were the sole means by which she could obtain relief. At consultation a perilous condition indicating the presence of organic disease was evident, and a more carefully selected dietary, with the employment of the usual natural hygienic accompaniments of treatment, was prescribed and faithfully carried out for six months. At the end of this time the patient, in full enjoyment of the relief that invariably appears in disease when organic labor is lessened by diet judiciously lowered, or by abstinence from food, insisted upon undergoing an absolute fast.

After three weeks, during which liquid food only was ingested, the total abstinence stage was entered, and the condition of the case visibly improved. On the twentieth day of fasting the patient decided for herself that her stomach could tolerate food. Experience demonstrates that persons who suffer from chronic disease after a time develop, as a consequence of repeated disappointment in search of health, a mental tendency that is willful, not to say stubborn. And in serious cases, such as the one under discussion, it is a question whether the better policy lies in acquiescence or in resistance to their expressed desires. In this instance no opposition was offered when the will to fast was expressed, nor was any attempted when the demand was now made for food. Because of structural organic deficiency, later fully discovered and then most evident in symptom, the digestive organs could not perform the tasks entailed, and ingestion of food resulted in nausea with vomiting, while hiccoughs in severe form, a sign most apprehensive in character, that in the circumstances indicated intestinal obstruction, occurred and continued intermittently until death intervened.

When a case exhibits in aggravated form the symptoms noted, and when, moreover, its history is one of prolonged suffering, it is a virtual certainty that extreme organic impairment exists that can in no wise be overcome. But, in order that no question might arise concerning the remedial agencies employed and in order to allay the distress of the family, the condition of the case was brought to the attention of several medical practitioners. They suggested a number of things, but none of their suggestions proved of avail, for unanimously they insisted upon feeding the woman, whose stomach was rejecting all forms of food, retaining even water with difficulty. The condition described continued for more than two weeks, with pulse and temperature at average normal, but with no visible improvement Again at the insistence of the family another consultation of medical doctors was called, its personnel consisting this time of three prominent specialists in intestinal disease. They concurred in the opinion that the patient was suffering from cancer of the stomach and pronounced the case as one without hope of recovery. In the latter respect they were right, for death came at the end of the fortieth day of abstinence from food.

The autopsy made known a condition which the symptoms had predicated. The stomach occupied a position in the abdominal cavity such that its pyloric opening was turned and held forward and downward six or seven inches from its normal position; the rounded portion of the lower center of the organ lay opposite the navel, and its shape was distorted and enlarged to a length of nearly two feet, and to a capacity of six fluid quarts. The small intestines were adherent at a number of points to the peritoneum, and the stomach also had to be released by the knife from the abdominal walls before it could be fully examined. The gall sac was excessively enlarged, while the liver was in a state of degeneration.

The medical history of this case notes typhoid fever with peritonitis about twelve years before death. This in all probability determines the time of causation of the visceral adhesions and of the distortion in stomach and intestines, for, when the typhoid symptoms occurred, the organs of the body of the patient were fully matured, and the inflammation incident to the symptoms, with constant feeding even while fever was at its height, gave no opportunity for the healing processes of nature to act. This combination of error eventually led to the formation of the lesions described, to which the fatal outcome is directly traceable.

It is perhaps unnecessary to emphasize the truth that, in the physical distress suffered by this woman, medicine was unable to grant her relief. In fact, the time when she was most free from suffering was covered by the last several weeks of fasting before death occurred.

During the forty days of abstinence large quantities of blackish offensive fluid was discharged with each enema, and there was progressive relief from distress with lessened pain. However, no decrease in the amount of refuse evacuated was noted until the power of function of the eliminative organs diminished with lowering vitality.

Case 2 is that of a married woman, thirty-nine years of age, who for all of the adult period of life had suffered greatly from impaired digestion, variously diagnosed by many different physicians. For two years prior to death the patient had subsisted upon a diet of liquid food, the stomach refusing solids. This woman since girlhood had the distinction of consistently refusing medical remedies, but, nevertheless, her condition steadily grew worse, and, while no hope was offered that recovery could be had, her request that she be permitted to undergo a fast was granted. No food, excepting the slight amount of nourishment contained in the juice of oranges and lemons in small quantities was given for fifty-seven days, when she died. In fact, at no time from the beginning of the fast, which really was undertaken because the stomach repeatedly rejected the liquids ingested, could food have been introduced into the organ. This was absolutely determined by the results of the autopsy, which are now given.

In the duodenum, just below the pyloric opening of the stomach, there must at one time have been an ulcer or some acute inflammation. Nature in her efforts at repair had deposited tissue cells at this point to the degree that the lumen of the intestine had been almost occluded. As time went by this growth enlarged and involved the bile ducts, so that when death occurred the passage through the duodenum was entirely blocked. In composition the accumulation of tissue showed none of the characteristic cell formation of cancer, but was a mass of muscle and membrane, healthy in their components, but abnormal in deposition. The right kidney was in a state of complete degeneration, but the other organs of the body and the intestines, with the exception of the duodenal portion, were normal in size, position, and condition.

In view of the remarkable circumstances involving the physiology of this woman, a fuller description of her dietetic habit proves interesting. As stated, for two years previous to death only liquids were tolerated. Food substances obtained by boiling vegetables and by diluting fruit juices were the forms in which sustenance was furnished. In fact, so intolerant of solids was the stomach that the broths and juices were strained through cloths in order that no formed particles entered into them. Whenever the straining was defective, vomiting of sediment occurred, hence the utmost care was needed so that distress might not be caused.

This case, then, subsisted for two years upon only that sustenance which her body was able to appropriate through stomach absorption. Mineral salts and the vitamins may conceivably be conveyed in part to the centers of nutrition in this manner, but it could only have been in minute amounts that proteins, carbohydrates, and the starches were delivered, and then in forms not fully digested. While, until a year or so before her death, there might have been a small passage through and past the accumulation in the duodenum, thus permitting of some intestinal digestion, it is certain that months of existence had elapsed with no food ingested other than that described as strained

bowel receives the benefit of the flow, and dilatation of the rectum and flexure is almost certain to occur with possible structural injury.

When a patient is bedridden or is extremely weakened, the knee-chest posture or the right-side position may prove too difficult or too exhausting to assume. In either of these contingencies, when no specially constructed table is at hand, a canvas stretcher upon which the subject may lie can be placed over the bath tub. If this apparatus cannot be procured, a triangular platform of three foot-wide boards covered with oiled cloth and a blanket, its base arranged so as to cross the top of the tub beneath the buttocks, may be used as a substitute. By the means indicated all effort in maintaining position is removed, a matter of importance in states of excessive weakness.

The operator in administering the enema, or the patient himself, in order to insure full benefit, will find it necessary to repeat the injection until the fluid returns comparatively colorless. This may mean that as many as twenty quarts of water may be required to obtain the desired result. Of course this amount of water cannot be introduced into the bowel at one time, but the contents of one bag or can, preferably of three-quart capacity, can be injected in the ordinary case and then evacuated with its accompanying refuse, and this operation may then thereafter be repeated until cleansing of the bowel is assured. Repetition as described is most essential in employing the internal bath, since the injection of only a small quantity of water

internal bath.

Post mortem examination discovered the liver in an advanced condition of degeneration; the stomach exhibited an extreme hour-glass contraction, and its pyloric opening would not permit the insertion of a probe the size of a lead pencil, while the walls of its lumen were cirrhosed or hardened; the small intestines and the colon throughout their lengths displayed a series of cartilaginous contractions. These structural defects were undoubtedly developed after arrival at maturity, since the unaffected portions of the organs were normal in size and in condition. The fetus was removed from the uterus at the autopsy, and was found to be in excellent state, exhibiting the normal development of an unborn child at four months.

Case 4. This was a married woman of thirty-five years, and the case is similar in many respects to the one preceding. The patient fasted fifty-nine days from the beginning of illness until death. The entire adult life of this woman had been made wretched by digestive impairment, bilious attacks, and menstrual difficulties. Drugs, including patent medicines, had done their worst until about two years before death, when, in hopeless apathy, the patient consented to undergo a fast, and completed one of thirty days with such success that she experienced full relief from menstrual pain thereafter, and there was but little digestive distress unless there had been carelessness in diet.

The compelling cause that led to the second fast

lay in the organic condition, later discovered, that had progressed to the point that the digestive function became inoperative. Morbid degeneration of the liver must have existed for some time previous to the beginning of abstinence, for from the first day of the fast black bilious discharge in quantity discolored the fluid of the enemas. The condition gradually became so aggravated that the thought of food tended to produce nausea, while its odor and even the perfume of flowers could not be borne. Organic defect had without doubt been present when the first fast took place, for its symptoms were noted at that time, but the organs affected, recuperated to a degree by their enforced rest and assisted by general systemic purification, were enabled to continue partial functioning for some months longer.

In the second fast pulse and temperature rose above normal register several points each day, but fell to average standard after the internal bath, which in this case was administered twice daily.

As in the previous case pregnancy of some months complicated conditions. On the fifty-first day of abstinence it was discovered that contractions of the uterus were occurring, and in a short while, with some manual assistance, a dead, misshapen fetus was delivered with little or no distress or pain. General relief was immediate, and it was so pronounced as to inspire the family with hope of ultimate recovery; but the improvement was succeeded by a decline in vitality that ended in the death of the patient.

During the latter days of this fast hiccoughs in severe form were present, and there was some vomiting of blackish bile. It was useless to attempt feeding at any stage of the fast, for, from the first, the stomach refused even water, and the only manner in which the fluids of the body were renewed was through absorption from the baths, both external and internal.

Post mortem findings follow. The liver was so degenerated that but little functioning could have occurred for many days; the gall sac was at least four times its normal in size and contained foul, black, bilious fluid; the kidneys were hypertrophied or enlarged, and pocketed with pus; the pancreas was so hardened in texture as to resist the knife; the spleen was degenerated to the degree that the organ was held together merely by its surrounding membrane; the small intestines were normal in size, condition, and position, as was the colon, excepting that the transverse portion of the latter organ had suffered malposition and in portions was no larger in diameter than the adult thumb; the right ovary contained a cyst filled with fluid, while the right fallopian tube was bent twice upon itself; the left ovary was in an atrophic or wasted state and was no larger than a lima bean in size; the heart and the lungs were normal.

Case 5 is that of a young man of twenty-five who had been syphilitically infected five years before death, and who had had his symptoms treated by medical practitioners and by advertising quacks. At the time of consultation syphilitic sores still remained, and other evidences of the blood taint were present. There was a loss of mental control that necessitated constant attendance of a nurse. About six months before death a fast of twenty-eight days was undertaken and successfully finished. At its completion the syphilitic sores had entirely disappeared, and relief in general was such that the patient was enabled to dispense with his attendant and to care for himself. But several months later signs of serious organic breakdown, including loss of mental control, again were apparent. One of the symptoms noted was that of copious discharge of watery mucus from the nasal passages and throat, together with constant, profuse exudation of sweat about the face and head. The latter symptom was present in such degree that the hair of the patient dripped moisture continuously and his pillow needed change every hour. Considerable solid feces and catarrhal mucus appeared in the enemas, and for a month before death speech was impossible and no function could be performed without assistance. No food was given during the last nineteen days of life.

Post mortem findings showed a brain, the right hemisphere of which was much degenerated and pus laden; the left hemisphere was structurally normal; the right jugular vein was occluded with a whitish deposit, not analyzed; the heart was normal; the right lung was in a state of embolism, and was virtually a mass of clotted blood, useless for its purposes; the left lung was normal; the liver was partially degenerated. In this case no abnormality existed throughout the length of the alimentary canal, and the kidneys, pancreas, and spleen were in condition that presumed ability to function.

Case 6, that of a man forty-six years of age, presents a history of constant disease with intermittent acute crises. As the result of an accident in childhood, by which the subject was injured internally, both youth and early manhood were punctuated with a succession of severe illnesses, which were treated in orthodox: without permanent relief. About fifteen years before death the patient abandoned medicine and turned to natural therapeutics, with the result that the first lengthy relief from physical distress was obtained. Three years before he died, acute disease again appeared, and, because of uncongenial but unavoidable environment, medical treatment was resorted to for a short time, again without benefit. Reverted to in finality, the fast and its accompaniments succeeded in relieving conditions to the extent that the patient was enabled to resume his wonted work. Although he suffered at intervals from this time on, there was no return of acute distress until the month preceding death, when, after somewhat strenuous exercise followed by a heavy meal, severe intestinal pains developed. For thirty days no food was given, the stomach rejecting even water, and at the end of the period named, virtually in constant pain the while, the patient died.

Post mortem examination showed an organic condition that was most abnormal. The lungs were adherent to the walls of the pleural cavity and to the diaphragm; the heart was slightly enl arged but functionally capable; the stomach was dilated and prolapsed; the gall sac was divided into three distinct pouches, two of which were filled with a total of one hundred and twenty-six stones, ranging in size from that of a pea to one four inches in circumference; the small intestines were collapsed and midway in their lower portion were intussuscepted so that two yards of their length were telescoped into but five inches, and here the diameter of lumen was only one-quarter of an inch; all of the small intestines were below normal in size; the transverse colon lay in front of the descending part of the bowel, an abnormality which largely increased the labor of disposing of body waste; the ascending and descending portions of the colon were lacking in development and were cirrhosed or hardened in structure; the sigmoid bend and the rectum were of diameter not to exceed that of an adult thumb, and were in an advanced state of cirrhosis; the liver, the pancreas, and the spleen all exhibited partial atrophy; brain and nerve centers showed no signs of deterioration.

As has been stated, surgical intervention is at times essential in order to correct accidental or congenital structural defect in tissue, and here was a case in which such intervention might have been successfully invoked at the time of the accident noted in its history. Neglected then, life was nevertheless prolonged despite the handicap of the abnormalities described, but at cost constant suffering.

Case 7, that of a man fifty-six years of age, presents

a history of continuous disease in youth, but includes at least twenty years of adult life devoted to corrective dieting, judicious fasting, and to constant hygienic care of the body. At the time that the case was brought to the attention and placed under the direction of the writer, the patient was aware that his condition was such that recourse must be had to every agency promising relief or he must succumb. After examination, the symptoms showing marked organic irregularities, it was agreed that but one hope of prolonging life remained, and that this lay in an absolute fast. By it would be determined either the ability of the organism to continue functioning, or assurance that the human machine had reached the point where life could be no longer maintained.

The fast began, and there was no marked disturbance until the twenty-first day, while relief was such that the patient and all about him hoped and believed that the improvement noted was permanent in character; but on this day and thereafter unfavorable symptoms progressively developed, and on the thirty-second day of the fast, the case lapsed into coma, which continued until an abscess which had formed in the nasal cavity was with difficulty discharged. Great ease in all respects resulted, and the patient became conscious, assisting with interest in the efforts being made to promote his recovery. Death, however, occurred on the thirty-eighth day of fasting.

At all times during this fast large amounts of mucus were discharged in the enemas, and at intervals pain, sometimes excruciating in kind, was felt in the bladder. In the latter stages pus in abundance appeared in the urine, and during the last few days of life the bladder ceased functioning, its contents being removed by catheterization. In this case muscular strength was shown in remarkable degree, during the fast and until the day of death. The patient was able at all times during consciousness to move himself in bed, to rise at intervals, and to assist himself in ways that seemed marvelous when his condition is considered.

The following are the results of the autopsy. The brain, weighing forty-eight and one-half ounces, was perfect in structure. Here again is corroborative evidence of the truth advanced by Dr. E. H. Dewey, and developed by all who have scientifically investigated and practically applied the fast as a therapeutic measure, viz., that nerve tissue is never depleted during abstinence, since its supply of sustenance is gained directly from body reserve, not from material freshly assimilated and appropriated by cells other than those of nerve substance. The lungs of this man were in excellent condition; the heart, organically considered, was perfect, but was filled with a gelatinous mass of serum affected by post mortem change; from the cardiac opening of the stomach to within two inches of the pylorus there was not a particle of healthy membrane, and the appearance of the walls of this organ was that of smooth, wet chamois skin; the duodenum was below normal in size, the upper portion of the jejunum being, however, somewhat dilated; about midway in the tube of the small intestine a downward intussusception had taken place, in length about two and one-half inches; this was of long-standing, since the walls of the bowel had become hardened and thickened, and thus the opening through the gut had been considerably reduced; the only section of the colon that was in normal state was the cecum, and thence to the rectum the organ was infantile in size; in fact, there was not an inch of this part of the intestinal tract into which the tip of the index finger could have been introduced; the sigmoid flexure was less developed than any other portion of the gut; in reality it was not a flexure or bend, being merely a straight vertical canal continuing the descending colon to the rectum and anus; the liver was much congested, its left lobe, however, being partly cirrhosed; the gall bladder was distended with bilious fluid; the pancreas was much undersize, and the spleen was that of an infant; the kidneys were in a state of degeneration and were pocketed with pus, which discharged through the ureters into an inflamed bladder, which was itself undersize and capable of containing within its thickened walls barely three ounces of urine.

In connection with this undeveloped and functionally inadequate digestive tract, it is interesting to record that the sex organs of this man were those of a boy of twelve or thirteen. He was underweight and boyish in appearance as well. The condition met was of course the result of disease in early life with consequent arrest of organic development.

Case 9, a civil engineer, twenty-seven years of age,

had suffered since childhood with intermittent acute digestive disease, which was treated as is usual in orthodox practice. Malnutrition finally became so pronounced that the subject decided that medicine could no longer suggest anything to alleviate his condition, and he entered a fast of his own volition, coming for consultation some days after its beginning. Examination at this time showed the uselessness of attempting to cope with the organic symptoms that were most plainly apparent, and it was deemed best to inform the patient that recovery was out of the question. To allay as much as was possible the fears of his family, food was given, but the stomach persistently rejected it, and the fast was perforce continued. The patient died at the end of twenty-one days of abstinence.

Post mortem examination revealed an organism with heart, lungs, and digestive organs so extremely arrested in development that, had it not been for the adult body in which they had been functioning, they would have been considered as the organs of a child four years of age.

Case 10, a man of thirty-four, whose physical history had been one of constant illness after his twentieth year, is next presented. The patient had been treated medically for indigestion, constipation, and for various fevers. All his life he had been a heavy meat eater and an inveterate user of strong tea. In later years fermentation, difficulty in breathing, and abdominal pain invariably succeeded the ingestion of a meal. For the relief of these symptoms medical correctives and tonics were taken, but the condition gradually grew worse. The patient finally decided to try a fast, but, because of interference by his family, a liquid diet was substituted and continued for thirty-five days when death occurred. In this case pulse and temperature before the dietetic regimen began had been constantly below normal, and during the period given they showed but little change, the pulse standing at fifty-four or thereabouts, with temperature as low at times as ninety-three.

The autopsy disclosed the lungs completely filled with an exudation of serous fluid, a condition that was the immediate cause of death. The surface of the body for several weeks had been discolored in spots, these blotches, or cyanosed areas, indicating an obstructed circulation. This symptom is sometimes present in cases of cirrhosis of the liver, and the latter organ was found in an advanced stage of atrophic hardening. The stomach held but eight fluid ounces, and it could hold no more, for its outside muscular coat was in a permanent state of contraction, while its mucus membrane was very much thickened, making the walls of the organ at least one inch in depth or thickness. As a result of the contraction of the outside coating of the stomach, it had become elongated into a tube, and its normal capacity was much diminished. The duodenum and the upper three feet of the small intestine were dilated so that their lumen was three inches in diameter, a structural change which suggests the thought that nature had attempted to remedy in this portion of the alimentary canal the deficiency in size and function existing in the stomach. It is said that cirrhosis of the stomach is a symptom very rarely observed in disease, but in this case and in the one that follows, this organic change was present in forms that could scarcely have been more perfect examples of their kind. Continuing the post mortem findings, below the dilated section of the small intestines the remainder of the tract including the entire colon was apparently normal in size and in functional ability. The gall bladder was small, while the kidneys, the pancreas, and the spleen all exhibited signs of tissue hardening.

Case 11, an unmarried woman of thirty-three, had never passed a year during infancy and girlhood free from acute illness, and had been a sufferer through all of her later life from nervous exhaustion that at frequent intervals was accompanied with morbid craving for food, a desire which was satisfied without reason whenever it occurred. About five years before death the medical adviser of the patient ordered that she take some sustenance every two hours during her waking moments, with a full meal just before retiring. In addition to her other suffering, for many years at the menstrual period, the young woman was compelled to lose four or five days from her duties. She had sought the world over for relief, and about two years before consultation had turned to natural agencies for health restoration undergoing then a fast of ten days. At the time the case was presented for examination there could be no doubt but that some aggravated form of organic disease existed, and no encouragement was offered in prognosis, but it was agreed that the treatment given should be aimed at the relief that a light diet, coupled with the essential eliminative accessories, would be certain to afford. This course was pursued for a period of eighty days, when death occurred. The case when first seen showed a cyanosed condition of the skin; the cheeks were blue and veined, as was the nose, and the entire surface of the body exhibited deplorable deficiency in venous circulation. This state improved to some extent after entering upon the dietary regimen.

Examination of the body after death revealed a liver and stomach cirrhosed, the stomach walls showing no evidence of recent function, being approximately three-quarters of an inch in thickness. The small intestines, infantile in size, were of the consistency of cartilage in sections, and adhesions were present at various points. The colon was no larger than an adult thumb throughout its length, and it also exhibited adhesions. The only organs of the body that were in anything like a condition of functional capability were the lungs and the heart. The kidneys, the spleen, and the pancreas, as in the previous case, were incipiently hardened.

In several of the cases quoted it has been mentioned that the patient after the beginning of a fast, experienced a renewal of vitality for which no solid physiological foundation existed. Nature, struggling to restore organic function, invariably makes the effort commensurate with the gravity of the existent defect. By the removal of the labor of digestion at least one-half of the total organic work of the body is lifted, and relief that simulates recuperation is manifested despite structural deficiency in the machine. In the presence of serious organic disease this seemingly favorable symptom is of short duration, and, as it passes, very evident decline begins and progresses until nerve centers and brain no longer receive adequate support and the body dies. In Cases 3 and 4 the relief experienced after the first fast was sufficient in each case, with organs still partially able to function, to enable the system to maintain itself until accumulation again became too great to permit of continuance. Defects in organism, too serious to have been corrected in the earlier treatment or in the interim, now reached the stage either of degeneration or of atrophy, until finally liberation of the life principle became no longer possible.

When a case is first presented for examination the presence of serious organic defect cannot always be determined, but no doubt is permitted shortly after entrance into a fast, for within a week or ten days symptoms are displayed that fix conditions. The third week positively decides the outcome. In the two cases last described signs of organic disease were such as not to be mistaken from the very first. Soon or late the result in these and like instances must be death, and all that can be done towards possible recovery must in the circumstances prove of no avail. Because of the hopeless outlook the cases described were placed upon restricted diet; a diet that put no undue strain upon failing function, but that, nevertheless, did not ameliorate the distress of disease as would an absolute fast. Family anxiety and outside criticism prevented the employment of the latter agency. In the circumstances life was prolonged for several weeks, but it is virtually certain that, if food had been entirely excluded, relief would have been greater and days would have been added to existence.

Disease that is functional in character is self-limited. The amount of poison manufactured within the body is determined by the intake of food or of drugs, and eradication of disease is fixed in limit of time by the ability of vital organs to resist and east out toxic products. The possibility always exists that these organs may prove unequal to their work, and this possibility becomes a certainty, with death as the outcome, in two situations—one, when the organs themselves are structurally defective, and the other, when, though fully capable of normal function, their powers are stimulated by food or by drugs, or by both, to the point of exhaustion. But one of these conditions, that of irreparable organic defect, presents itself when disease is treated by means of the fast. Both are encountered in the therapeutics of medicine.

In the majority of instances in medically treated cases the passing of life occurs under the influence of opiates that deaden pain and paralyze consciousness. Virtually from the beginning of a fast pain ceases, consciousness is usually maintained with exceptional mental clarity, and death, if it occurs, is like falling into gentle sleep.

The results displayed in the post mortem findings cited, and the comparisons made in the statement that follows, are tangible assets in the claim that, in the absence of defects in the organs of the body, abstinence from food, together with the needful health-giving and health preserving accompaniments elsewhere described in the text, is the unfailing remedy for the correction of functional ills. Both physician and patient from the outset of treatment possess the assurance of recovery; and confidence that rests on infallible natural law is in itself of the greatest assistance in accomplishing results.

Comparative statement of post mortem findings is death by starvation (medical), and post mortem findings in death during the fast as noted in the text.